THE ROAD TO WEIGHT LOSS

CREATE YOUR ROADMAP TO WEIGHT LOSS SUCCESS

OLIVER JAMES

Copyright © 2024 Oliver James Smith

All rights reserved.

No part of this publication may be reproduced, stored in a retrieval system or transmitted in any form or by any means, without the prior permission in writing of the publisher, nor be otherwise circulated in any form of binding or cover other than that in which it is published and without a similar condition including this condition being imposed on the subsequent purchaser.

ISBN: 9798325233265

The information in this book is not intended to replace or conflict with the advice given to you by your GP or other health professionals. All matters regarding your health should be discussed with your GP. The author disclaims any liability directly or indirectly from the use of the material in his book by any person.

DEDICATION

To You.
For deciding to follow a different road to others.
I admire that.

CONTENTS

	About The Author	7
	Introduction	11
1	Why Weight Loss Is Hard	31
2	Understanding Body Weight	63
3	The Elephant And The Rider	83
4	Track Your Food Intake	107
5	Grow Yourself	129
6	Bright Spots	193
7	Find The Feeling	203
8	Shrink The Change	227
9	Script The Critical Moves	237
10	Point To The Destination	249
11	Shape The Road	277
12	Ride Into The Sunset	303

ABOUT THE AUTHOR

I'm not too fond of these things as they tend to be an opportunity for the author's ego to grow—a moment of self-indulgence and showing off in the hope of proving credible to the reader. I always read them and think they're false. Not many people walk around telling everyone how good they are at something or how qualified they are for a role. This isn't an interview. It's also not a self-absorbed section where I tell you to put me on a pedestal and kiss my feet. I'm not arrogant, so I'm certainly not going to begin my book like that. Instead of the peacocking, it should be as if we were meeting in person.

When you first meet someone, you introduce yourself: "Hi, I'm Oliver from The Weight Loss Academy". You do the formalities: "I'd like to thank you for trusting me to help you lose weight by showing you the road to weight loss. Working together, we will create your weight loss roadmap. I won't let you down.". Then you get to know each other a little. "This is a little awkward as you can't speak back. I believe you wish to lose weight, and I'd like to get to know you better. You can introduce yourself in the Weight Loss Academy forum at www.theweightlossacademy.com/join. This is where each

ABOUT THE AUTHOR

person who reads this book can introduce themselves and share their story. I want to build a community, and the more we know about each other, the more we can all help and support one another.

I live in Manchester, UK, and I've been a weight loss coach since 2009. I've always enjoyed playing sports, but over the years, my body hasn't, and I'm more of a spectator now. I describe myself as a normal guy, but I suppose we all do, don't we? I'm healthy but not obsessive. I eat well, most of the time. I love a bit of Tapas and a good pick and mix. I can be found on a spin bike but also on a series binge. I love all animals, a country walk and a good pub lunch. Can you tell me more about yourself?"

I always think people don't care how much you know until they know how much you care. You couldn't care less about my qualifications or experience. Nobody has ever asked me in my years as a weight loss coach, which says a lot. Nobody cares about the certificates I've collected and stored under my bed. They want to know how I can help them succeed on their weight loss journey. They want to know who I am as a person to see if we are a good fit for each other. They want to know how much I care.

I pride myself on being my own person. This carries into my career, where I do things my own way. I'm not bothered by what everybody else is doing. I have a way of working with people and helping them lose weight that is different as it puts the person first. I don't encourage each person I work with to live the same life as me. I provide

ABOUT THE AUTHOR

them with the mentoring and support needed to make their own decisions in life.

Let's not reinvent the bloody wheel. A wheel has been circular since the 4th millennium BC, so I can't see it changing to a triangle, even if Elon Musk is sending people to live on Mars. I can safely say that even with this possibly happening in my lifetime, I can't see a wheel changing to a triangle any time soon, can you? If that's the case, why are we trying to reinvent weight loss every five seconds? Too many cooks in the kitchen? Too many egos? In a world where things are accessible, we appear to have diluted the wisdom, overlooked the basics, and steered off in the wrong direction.

I suppose it's the same as sending people 300 Million miles off on a rocket at 24,600 mph to live on Mars when we could look after the planet we live on. Plus, it would take nine months to get there. Who's got the patience to spend nine months stuck on a rocket to end up at a baron landscape of red rock? At least when you spend nine months losing weight, you won't be confined or restricted. Instead, you will have the freedom to explore and enjoy the journey. Once you get there, you will be happy with the destination, looking in the mirror at the person you've always dreamed of being.

I'm not a know-it-all. Nobody knows all the answers, and those who claim they do know nothing. What I do know is you've come to the right place. I help people achieve their goals. This is your weight loss journey, and I will use my knowledge and experience to help you. Once again, I thank you for putting your trust in me. I respect you

ABOUT THE AUTHOR

for taking a different approach to the common ways of losing weight. I appreciate you for reading this book. I won't let you down. Follow The Road To Weight Loss.

Oliver

INTRODUCTION

Weight loss can be hard. It can be challenging to achieve. And let's face it; it can be boring chomping on healthy food when everyone else is having a good time. I'm never going to deny these three statements as they're true. They are beliefs most of us have concerning weight loss. At the same time, you can believe the road to weight loss can be simple, straightforward, and enjoyable. I felt the need to write a book as I'm sick and tired of people feeling trapped, frustrated, and like a failure. I feel compelled to show you the road to weight loss can be direct. It doesn't have to consist of winding roads, which are full of roadblocks and getting lost. It can be simple to achieve. Weight loss isn't as hard as you think.

Although you don't get paid for it, weight loss is work. It's not a hobby, even though many people like to jump from one weight loss method to another in the same way they switch from series to series on Netflix. Nobody will say losing weight when you ask people about their hobbies. Yet, at the same time, people seem to love talking about it. People congregate in the playground, the slimming club, or the gym studio and

INTRODUCTION

share their views, results, and advice. We have so much information from many angles that it's hard to differentiate between beneficial and superficial. Lost in the noise around us is the proven truth about weight loss. It's the result of the realisation there is a simple way of losing weight. You know there must be a way, so you've been searching for one for a while. Now you've found it to solve a problem that's been around for years: How do I lose weight?

If you purchased this book, assuming I had a magic wand, please stop reading and get a refund. This book isn't about who can lose weight the quickest. It's about who can lose weight the most efficiently. The quick fix has caused us to have false expectations on various weight loss methods. I can't lose the weight for you. You've got to put in the work, which is why you must approach your weight loss journey as though you're going to work. You don't get paid to do nothing so why would you think you can achieve your weight loss goal without putting in a little effort? You must read this book, take action at the end of each chapter, and remain consistent when following the roadmap you create. Don't get me wrong, I will show you the most streamlined road to weight loss, but this still requires thinking for yourself, motivation, and perseverance.

Weight loss is a choice. A choice you've made that's brought you here today. Achieving your weight loss goal is not an order from somebody else. It's the desire to achieve it which must be done your way. This book is for those who wish to take control, achieve, and

INTRODUCTION

flourish, not those who only dream. It's for those who want to make a dream their reality. The people who have achieved their weight loss goal live in a reality you have only ever dreamed of. It would help if you found the courage to believe in your ability, as this is when the fun begins. You can never cross the ocean unless you dare to lose sight of the shore. Do you believe in yourself, or is the fear of failure keeping you pinned to the shoreline? The fear of losing weight only to gain it again. The fear of slipping up, embarrassing yourself and starting again. Get your toes wet. Who cares what anybody thinks? Your life isn't yours if you constantly care what others think.

Our weight loss journeys are based on compliance with the rules set out by the diet industry. They are a wolf in sheep's clothing as they don't wish you to succeed. We trust them to give us what we need, yet they give us a glimmer of success, only to have it snatched back off us. They lead you to consume their products and obey their rules. To lose weight, you must go on a specific diet and do as they say. When you fail to keep the weight off, you must blame yourself, not them. Once you've stopped being upset about your failures, you must grovel back to them to 'help' you again. This formula has been with us since William Banting's Letter on Corpulence in 1863. He is also known for being the first to popularise a weight loss diet based on limiting the intake of carbohydrates. Since then, more and more people have followed suit and told us what we can and can't do. It's time to take

INTRODUCTION

the shackles off and stop blaming yourself. Instead, you can create your own way of eating, consume the foods you choose to eat, and comply with rules set out by yourself.

Setting your own rules and following a different route to others is inherently scary. This journey is one without an external saviour. You must trust yourself to be the unique human you are. Make decisions that are in your best interest, no matter what others say or do. It's better to follow your own road imperfectly than to follow someone else's perfectly. As you continue down the road to weight loss, you will gain confidence in your ability, be accountable for yourself, and learn as you go. It's a journey of growth both inside and out. As others stop, you continue. Creating your roadmap requires energy to think and a contribution from one's self. It's a holistic approach to weight loss, taking on board all factors that affect weight. If you look at each person who has made it to their destination, their routes will differ, but the structure of their journey is the same. You are in charge. Trust yourself. I'm solely here to provide the structure to your journey by helping you create your weight loss roadmap.

There's a way of losing weight that works for all. It's not a diet; it's a structure to your life. This structure allows something complex to become simple to achieve. For too long now, we've been sweating the small stuff and focusing on the things that don't matter. Weight loss isn't achieved when focusing on one specific thing; it's all things. There comes a time when

INTRODUCTION

you must step back. When you do this, you see the bigger picture. It would be best to ensure the essential things are not being pushed out of the way by the seemingly urgent need of the moment.

A roadmap is a long-term plan showing you how something is arranged to accomplish your goal. It's goal-setting, change-making, and action-taking. It factors in all parts of your life to ensure you stand the best possible chance of success from your lifestyle, environment, feelings, and personality. A roadmap ensures you achieve your weight loss goal. As you create your roadmap, you will be encouraged to take action. You must embrace the process of self-improvement and understand that enjoying the journey is as important as arriving at the destination. Writing words on paper is not a roadmap. It doesn't matter how pretty your roadmap looks or who has the best one. What matters is that the words you write on paper spark something in your mind, and action is taken. You must understand that actions are all we can control. This roadmap is simply the beginning of your future. You will venture down the road to weight loss and at some point, these actions will get results.

The principles, structure and knowledge I share in this book will give you a stress-free, happy, and fulfilling weight loss journey. When your friends and family notice your excellent results and ask how you've done it, they will expect to hear of sacrifice, unhappiness, sweat and tears. You're used to telling them how hard you've been working. You want to

INTRODUCTION

impress them by telling them how hard it's been for you. But this time's different.

You know you can't stick to it. Deep down, you know there's nothing impressive about losing a few pounds through hard work and sacrifice, only to put back on the weight you've just lost. Once you've read this book and taken the actions I have instructed you to take, you will know that weight loss isn't as hard as you think. You will realise that it's a relatively simple process. When people ask you how you've managed to lose weight this time and keep it off, you can proudly look them in the eye and say, "I lost weight; it was straightforward and effortless, and I will never need to lose weight again." They may not sound impressed with the simplicity of your response, but you know that simplicity is the ultimate sophistication.

My promises to you

Before guiding you through the process that will help you lose weight, I must outline my four promises. The last thing I want is for you to waste your time reading a book that doesn't sound like it will help you.

I will get straight to the point

After your health, time is the most valuable thing. You live in a busy world. You have to go to work, make time for loved ones, slot in a bit of socialising with your friends, nip to the shops, do some jobs around the

INTRODUCTION

house, and now you're trying to squeeze in a casual bit of weight loss too! You've committed four and a half hours in your busy life to reading my book, which is a wise investment if I say so myself. I will ensure you won't waste any time following those ghastly weight loss gimmicks ever again. I don't need to make this book any longer than it needs to be. Everything within it serves a specific purpose. The last thing I want to do is drag you through pages and pages of content with very little substance.

Statistically, not everyone will complete reading this book. It's a fact, unfortunately, which is why I've written this book in order of most importance. Don't skip chapters, as you will miss essential information and actions. I was tempted to write stories for each chapter to show client scenarios as storytelling is an effective tool for learning; however, including stories would increase the size of the book, doubling the time it would take for you to read it. I've streamlined this book to ensure as many people as possible make it to the end. The higher the completion rate, the more people will lose weight. Could you make sure you're one of them?

I will be honest

Unfortunately, the weight loss industry is full of pork pies. People want to be different and stand out. They wish to be known as pioneers, gurus, or influencers. To stand out from the crowd, they must tell lies, some

INTRODUCTION

big and some small. Misinformation increases in the world of weight loss due to this. If one person tells you carbohydrates are bad, the next feels the need to sound different and tell you fats are bad. None of them are bad, by the way. Weight loss is a simple concept; however, once one person tells the world it's tricky, everyone thinks it's tricky. Remember when everyone rushed off to buy toilet paper during Covid? It only took one person in one country to start the panic, and before you know it, the whole world is rushing off to the supermarket. Diets are the same; it only takes one person in one country to start a new diet, and before you know it, the whole world follows it. Diets belong exactly where toilet paper belongs: down the drain.

I couldn't care less about being a pioneer or standing out. Yes, my methods are different to the weight loss diets out there; I wouldn't have felt the need to write a book otherwise. My methods are more about a way of living than a wacky weight-loss diet. A method is a particular procedure for accomplishing or approaching something. A diet is a specific course of food to which a person restricts themselves to lose weight. My methods provide structure and actions, and the dietary advice I share with you can be found in many other publications. You see, genuine dietary advice doesn't change; false information does. Everyone is out there searching for new dietary advice when, instead, the answers are already right in front of them. We've only been struggling with our weight over the past fifty years. What do you think has changed

INTRODUCTION

over the years to cause our weight issues to spiral out of control?

I will keep it simple

There's nothing worse than confusing names, fancy lingo, and heavy science books. You're reading this book to achieve one thing: to achieve your weight loss goal. I'm here to accomplish one thing: to show you it's not as hard as you think. Although I will need to cover some basic sciency stuff to help you down the road to weight loss, I will keep it simple. Yes, I may need to use words such as Leptin and Ghrelin, but I will explain them so it makes sense to you. If spell check wants to change the word Ghrelin to gremlin, it's confusing lingo.

I'm not here to impress you with big words. They don't help you move further down the road to weight loss. Suppose I need to use some fancy jargon, such as thermogenesis. In that case, I will use words or phrases you're more familiar with, such as metabolism. Although some health professionals will disagree with what I've just said, I don't care. I'm here to help you lose weight, and to do that, I need to keep it simple by using words or phrases you will easily understand.

I've outlined this book in a way that is simple to follow. The first part explains why you think weight loss is hard to achieve and helps you understand body weight. The rest provides a structure showing that weight loss isn't as hard as you think. Chapter by chapter, you will begin to see the road to weight loss is pretty straightforward. You will find to-do lists at the end of each part or chapter that encourage you to create a plan or take a particular action. The to-do lists ensure action is taken to move you further down the road to weight loss. Words are powerful because they can inspire action. But without action, words are just meaningless. Read the words, take action, and you will achieve your weight loss goal. It's that simple!

My requests to you

It would be best if you didn't go through the motions. I want you to commit to a brighter future. When working with clients in person, I ensure they commit to their journey by signing my six requests. If people don't commit, they will dip in and out, get confused, and be stuck in the diet trap for the rest of their lives. This may sound over the top; I assure you it is not. Without the commitment to a particular way, you will venture down the wrong road, weight loss will be difficult, and your weight will slide back and forth. With commitment, you will get your head down, realise weight loss is a simple process, and make it to your destination. These six requests are just as important as the content in the book.

1. Hold yourself accountable
2. Be patient with your journey

INTRODUCTION

3. Be clear on which road you're taking
4. Don't overcomplicate the process
5. Don't strive for perfection
6. If you don't know, ask

Hold yourself accountable

Without accountability, you have nothing. You could have all the information you need, the structure to succeed and the best coach in the world, yet you won't get anywhere if you don't hold yourself accountable. This is why it's my first request. You must call yourself out when you aren't doing things correctly, not negatively, but in a caring way. Accountability isn't about blaming yourself. It's about being responsible for your actions, and there's a big difference. Negative perceptions don't get you anywhere, as emotions dictate your direction. Accountability is a way to look after yourself and is the only way you will achieve anything in life. It's too easy to say, "Fuck it, it's Friday", and that's fine occasionally. Still, if it keeps happening, you must admit it and understand it's preventing you from achieving your goal.

We like to follow strict diets because we can blame them for not losing weight. We hire weight loss professionals to pass the buck on to them, "It's their responsibility now". This is not how it works. Yes, many shoddy diets are out there, and some weight loss' professionals' are talking out their rear end, but you are responsible for your actions. We all have times when we slip up; however, the difference between someone who achieves their weight loss goal and someone who doesn't is the speed at which one admits they slipped up, brushes themselves off and gets back on track.

In this book, you will create a framework and decide on the best course of action for you, then ensure you remain consistent with these actions. You decide your goals, which changes to make, the foods to eat and whether you do any activity. I put the power in your hands, and with it comes great responsibility. This can seem scary, but I will be with you every step of the way. Plus, it will be empowering when you begin to follow your own route. Do you agree to hold yourself accountable?

Be patient with your journey

You're enthusiastic and can't wait to work your way through this book and take action. This is your time to shine. Motivation runs through your veins, but how long will it last? Apologies, I know it's your time to shine, but I need to rain on your parade. You don't have an infinite amount of motivation. It runs out at some point, which is when most people stop trying to lose weight even though they want to. You can't solely rely on motivation to help you achieve your weight loss goal. You must play the long game and develop a structure for your weight loss journey, a roadmap to success. It's pointless losing weight quickly only to

INTRODUCTION

regain it; you know it's true. Reading this book, creating your weight loss roadmap, and taking action takes time. Don't get ahead of yourself by speeding through this book and taking many premature actions. I need you to slow yourself down for a second and encourage you to be patient with your journey. You will get results once it is sustainably possible.

I'm sure you would love to lose weight quickly. You may be used to seven pounds in seven days, dropping a dress size in a week, maybe even more, however, these are unrealistic expectations. These are marketing tactics to make you believe they are attainable. You've got to approach your weight loss with the mentality of losing one pound, never to gain that same pound back. Your big weight loss goal doesn't have to be achieved with a big, outlandish solution. Big goals are achieved with small, achievable changes that fit into your lifestyle. Keep it simple, be patient, and focus on making just one change at a time. Even though you're motivated to try and do more than I ask, don't. You won't be able to keep it up. Impatience is the biggest killer of progress. Do you agree to be patient on your weight loss journey and not get ahead of yourself?

Be clear on which road you're taking

I'm about to send you down a different road than the one you're used to following. All your weight loss friends have ventured down a different road. One you're familiar with following yourself. They are following a shortcut to their destination, requiring restriction and filled with boredom. Their body and emotions can't stick to it, so this shortcut leads them to a dead end.

It would help if you were clear that you can't take the shortcut others are taking. It doesn't matter how quickly their results initially come. What matters is keeping the weight off. I've asked you to hold yourself accountable and be patient on your weight loss journey. These already guide you down a different road than the one you've previously taken. You're used to being told what to do without having to think for yourself. You're also used to being told to "GO GO GO", which makes me telling you to slow down and be patient sound alien to you. The shackles are off, and you can spread your wings. Your new road is one to be enjoyed.

Your new road will initially feel like it won't deliver as it's not difficult to follow. You're also the only person following it, as it's a route unique to you. You get to decide what to eat and what changes to make. There's no stress through your journey as everything is mapped out and controlled. The route will be clear, and it's empowering to know you will only ever have to make this journey once. Your body will love this route as it will receive everything it desires. You will experience positive emotions as you enjoy yourself, feel different, and see sustainable results. You yearn for stillness and tranquillity. In doing so, you will be

INTRODUCTION

clear this route you've created is the one for you. Are you clear on which road you're about to take?

Don't overcomplicate the process

We're all guilty of trying to do fancy things. Head to a gym, and you will find plenty of people doing exercises that aren't beneficial and should be left to the circus. They're doing things that look impressive to others. The "I know more than you because I'm doing a silly exercise" brigade is out in full swing. Instead, they should be doing the most efficient exercises that bring them the best results in the shortest amount of gym time. Instead, they've been caught up in the show and have ended up doing complicated and inefficient exercises. If you thought the world of exercise was complicated, we're screwed in the world of food, dieting, and nutrition. I've just used three different words for the same thing. See how easy it is to overcomplicate things?

Nutritional science has been on the rise over the past few decades, which is excellent. The more scientific research on the foods we eat, the better, but it can leave people scratching their heads. It's also opened the doors to scientific research that's been manipulated to make it sound like it's the solution to your weight loss problem. Think of the rise of the ketogenic diet. It talks about being in a state of ketosis. This metabolic state occurs when your body burns fat for energy instead of glucose. Although there is such a thing as ketosis, and it is possible to do, they're trying to rewrite the rulebook and change the fundamentals. They're overcomplicating the process, something you shouldn't do. Our body relies on glucose for energy, and it has for our whole life, so why change it now? It would be best if you also understood how severe this change to your lifestyle would be. To understand how making this change is unnecessary. It's not going to be a walk in the park, I'll tell you that.

We're striving for breakthroughs in weight loss, but we don't need to. Because people have struggled with their weight for some time, they believe the new way on the market is the solution. The fundamental principle of weight loss has already been studied and confirmed, and it's a relatively simple concept to grasp when explained well. It takes a lot of hard work to make something clear and simple. To truly understand the underlying challenges and develop graceful solutions. I've done all the studying and brainwork for you, so you don't have to. I thoroughly understand the fundamentals of weight loss, which has allowed me to disregard many parts that are not essential. I urge you not to overcomplicate the process so I can pass on what I know and ensure you lose weight for good. Do you agree not to overcomplicate the process?

Don't strive for perfection

If I made this book perfect, you would not be here reading it right now. There may be a typo or two, a

INTRODUCTION

smidgen of poor grammar, but does it matter? If I strived for perfection, this book would never have been released. I can always make further changes at a later date. My purpose is to help you achieve your weight loss goal. It's not to challenge Shakespeare, Austen, or Dickens. Your purpose is to lose weight and keep it off, but you won't achieve this if you strive for perfection. I can't knock enthusiasm or ambition; however, waiting for the stars to align will prevent you from progressing or even beginning. There is no perfect time to start, no perfect diet to transform your body, and no perfect exercise plan. You must understand that something done well is better than nothing perfectly done. We all live busy lives, and perfection is unattainable.

You decide to exercise five times a week, miss a session, beat yourself up about it and stop exercising altogether. Choose to 'eat clean', are offered a brownie, you take it, get frustrated with yourself and stop eating clean. These strict expectations of yourself prevent you from being consistent and create negative feelings. They send you in the opposite direction to the one you were expecting. One exercise session is better than none. 60% healthy eating is better than 20%. If you lose weight in three weeks but gain a pound in one, does that mean you haven't lost weight that month? You can achieve your weight loss goal without the need to be perfect. Making mistakes is normal and is an opportunity to learn and improve. Two workouts per week, every week, will get better results than five workouts in one week. It's a more realistic approach. Consistency gets results. Focus on being better rather than perfect. We must all strive to better ourselves, yet one thing we mustn't do is set unrealistic expectations of our actions. Do you agree not to strive for perfection?

If you don't know, ask

At school, I needed some clarification on things my teachers were explaining. They would ask, "Does anybody have any questions?" but because others didn't put their hand up and I'd draw attention to myself, I wouldn't ask. If Google were as good as it is today, I would've just googled it when I got home, but it wasn't. I would go into my exam, the question would come up, and to no surprise, I'd get it wrong. If only I'd dared to ask a question. I request you to ask. Don't be like me and fear asking; Fear not knowing.

A book speaks to the masses, meaning you must include information from which everyone will benefit. The only issue with this is that you can occasionally miss things that affect certain people. This book contains 99% of the information needed for 99% of the people reading it. Due to some people's circumstances, dietary needs, or medical history, I may not specifically cover their needs. If this is you, you will need to ask questions.

Each person begins with the same broad goal of wanting to lose weight and will achieve this goal, yet

INTRODUCTION

their journeys will differ. You are creating a roadmap specifically for you, created by you. That's the unique part of this book; it doesn't tell you what to do. You decide what's best for you. At times, you may doubt the decision you've made or be unsure of the best route to take. If this happens to you, don't feel lost and remain silent. Ask a question.

You may have a question regarding something in this book, which action to take or something I don't cover. Never feel silly for asking a question. What's silly is not asking a question you don't have the answer to. If you have any questions, please visit the members forum at www.theweightlossacademy.com/forum and ask away. I will answer every question, no matter how silly it may sound. I'm here to help. It's my job and the purpose of this book — Do you agree to ask a question if you ever feel unsure, stuck or confused?

1

WHY WEIGHT LOSS IS HARD

When people try to lose weight, they're usually tinkering with their eating habits and trying to be more active. They do things they feel they should be doing and stop 'bad' habits. They take behaviours they associate with losing weight, known as automatic behaviours. These behaviours have been ingrained in the diet culture for 50-odd years, but are these automatic behaviours that everyone keeps doing the right ones? Should we all cut back on the carbs, hit the gym, or join a slimming club? Do these methods work for all? Are they the right choice for you? Most people's weight loss behaviours are automated reactions to weight loss, which can be wrong for you, making weight loss hard. The road to weight loss becomes distorted.

Trying to lose weight is great. We all have to try things to get better at them, but to get better; we need to try the things we stand a chance at sticking to. If you hate gyms, you aren't going to go multiple times a week, even if you try. If you hate cutting carbs, you aren't going to stick to that diet or way of eating, even if you try. You may last a week or two, but eventually, you won't be able to stick to it. If you try to attend a slimming club but are already restricted on time, you aren't going to go, even if you try. It's these scenarios where you fail to stick to the automated dieting behaviours. Weight loss isn't difficult, but if you select the incorrect actions you're programmed into believing are essential, it will feel that way. Following the wrong road causes weight loss to feel hard.

When an individual can identify their style and tendencies, they possess the power to successfully navigate their own way to their weight loss goal. They find a way of losing weight that will work for them and their lifestyle, which is one empowering thing. In doing so, they allow weight loss to be achieved easily. This is what I will be helping you find in this book. Before I do this, I need to explain in greater detail why you think weight loss is hard to achieve. This way, you know where you've gone wrong in the past, which will prevent you from falling into the same traps and following the wrong road in the future.

Reason 1 - He who shouts the loudest gets heard (unfortunately)

We live in a noisy world. One full of people fighting to get our attention. A world that's been taken over by people who love the sound of their own voice. A study in 2021

WHY WEIGHT LOSS IS HARD

showed that 90% of Twitter posts were made by just 10% of Twitter users. They're always shouting, and we hear them, but that doesn't mean they're right. People who post their lives on Instagram love to be seen, and posting captions underneath influences our decisions, but does that mean we should be influenced? TV experts and journalists love to be heard. You don't tend to see shy people on TV, do you? They tell us how we should live, eat, and work out to live healthier lifestyles, but just because they're in the public eye, does that make them right?

Many people produce excellent, informative content for people wishing to lose weight and live a healthier lifestyle. Still, more often than not, they aren't the ones being heard. They're drowned out and diluted by the sheer volume of people discussing the same subject. Unfortunately, we live in a culture where the one who shouts the loudest or posts the most gets the most attention. It's quantity over quality these days, and they hold one of the most powerful things in life: your attention. Leading to us taking advice and information that may not necessarily be in our best interest. Just because they're being heard, it doesn't mean they're right.

It might sound like I'm telling you to ignore everyone other than myself. I'm not. That's not how I work. This book isn't about me; it's about you. It's about you achieving your weight loss goal. I couldn't care less if you don't remember the author. All you need to remember is the content and strategy within this book so you can keep control of your weight for the rest of your life. I want you to stop and consider where you source your health and weight loss information. Who are you influenced by? What do you read? Who do you follow on social media? Do you allow them to tell you what's best for you? If so, how's that working for you?

If you find yourself influenced by the words of the failing diet culture, you must cut the source off. It's not going to help you. Don't allow your mind to be influenced by those who shout the loudest. They're generally shouting due to incompetence or insecurities about their methods. The matter can be escalated when several people try to outcompete each other to prove they're right. To lose weight with ease and simplicity, you must think about who you're allowing in your ears. If you stop listening and trust yourself instead, you will discover a stillness in your life.

Reason 2 - We mirror other people's actions

As the old saying goes, imitation is the most significant form of flattery. When we set off to do something new, we tend to mirror the actions of others already doing it. If they are doing something in a certain way, that's the way to do it, right? If you stand still for a second and assess the situation, you will see those actions come from people shouting the loudest. This doesn't mean they're right, so should we mirror their actions? What you will find is that everyone is either pretending they know what they're on about or following actions without actually knowing why.

When you set off to lose weight, you will follow a diet you've seen work for Reese Witherspoon. When your friend mentions that a slimming club worked for them and you should go too, you do because if it worked for them, it would surely work for you. An Instagram influencer with your dream body posts multiple times a day telling you how to get a body like theirs; of course, you will purchase their exercise plan. You venture into the gym for the first time and see the women on the treadmill and the men in the weights section; you find your gender and stick with what they're doing. Another person tells you what you're doing is wrong and that you should follow the diet that worked for them instead, so you jump ship and sail off in a different direction. We all feel the need to be right. It's part of human nature. But often, this need is due to insecurity or ego. Just because somebody tells you to do something with conviction, it doesn't mean you should do it. Strong and wrong, is still wrong.

Mirroring other people's actions is also a natural instinct. It starts before you're even born, as an unborn baby's heartbeat mirrors the same rhythm as the mother's when in the womb. We then ate the foods our family ate, liked the same things as them, had the same views and even acted the same way. When trying to make friends at school, you mirrored their behaviours and claimed to like what they liked. Even as adults, we do it, and most of the time, we don't even realise that we're doing it. We tend to mirror those we like or are interested in, which signals that we are connected to that person in some way. We mirror body language, speech, facial expressions, and behaviours. Next time you speak to somebody, notice how many things you mirror.

Evolutionarily, we were part of a tribe. We mirrored other people's behaviours within our tribe to give us a sense of belonging, leading to specific accents and behaviours in certain parts of the UK. Tribes are a survival instinct, but concerning weight loss, they are preventing you from achieving your weight loss goal. If we split weight into tribes, you would have three groups - People who are overweight, people who are trying to lose weight, and people who are a healthy weight. Here's where the problem lies. When you decide you wish to lose weight, this will mean leaving the overweight tribe and joining the weight loss tribe. This can include friends or family members who don't want to lose weight. It means losing some social situations or behaviours with your tribe, which can be challenging to navigate and cause friction, especially if you live with them.

Instantly, you think, "What are the weight loss tribe doing?" and mirror their behaviours to gain a sense of belonging in your new tribe. You follow people on Instagram, speak to others trying to lose weight about their journey, and are tempted to join a slimming club. You mirror the diets they are on, do the exercises they do, and act the way they appear to act. Before you know it, you're stuck in a diet culture that doesn't seem to work, as the people you've been mirroring don't know how to lose weight correctly. Your old tribe wants you back, and it's much more fun with them, so you slide back and forth between each tribe. The reason why you find weight loss difficult is because you've been mirroring the wrong tribe.

When you wish to lose weight, you must mirror the behaviours of the people who are a healthy weight, not the people who are trying to lose weight. You can learn a lot from this group of people. You will find they don't worry too much about their weight, have no extreme restrictions on what or when they can eat, and don't talk much about their weight. They have acquired the correct actions and are running on autopilot. Creating your weight loss roadmap will allow you to develop these actions yourself. Instead of mirroring the diet culture's actions, you will replicate the actions of people who are a healthy weight. Begin to assess the healthy people around you. What is their relationship with food like? How active are they? What do they think about their bodies? What does a typical meal look like? Overall, what lifestyle do they live?

There is a broad range of people who are of a healthy weight, which is why I need to finish by confirming that if you are to mirror healthy people, make sure they are regular folk. Athletes and models are healthy people, yet you need to walk before you can run. Many people have impressive physiques, with plenty telling you how they eat, exercise, and live. You must acquire the basic skills of being healthy to ensure you control your weight for the rest of your life. Once you achieve this, you can decide to replicate an athlete's lifestyle, but don't run before you can walk. If you do, weight loss will be difficult to achieve.

Reason 3 - There's a lack of clear direction from the industry

The weight loss industry is like the Wild West. It's unruly and lawless, and nobody has any control over it. People within it can do and say whatever they want. They can sell snake oil and get away with it, tell you how to lose weight without any qualifications and show you how to do exercises without being able to do them correctly. It's a mess, which is why losing weight is hard. How are you supposed to head off to your weight loss destination when everyone puts signs up with arrows pointing in different directions? You're trying to navigate the route without a clear map, so you're bound to get lost. It's not your fault you're lost. There's a lack of clear direction from the industry.

The weight loss and weight management industry is reported to be worth $251.51 billion annually. Yet, at the same time, obesity is rising rapidly, with an estimated 1.9 billion adults worldwide being classed as overweight, of which 650 million are classed as obese. The industry is failing us all, and they're doing it intentionally. Would you give up $251.51 billion? The more people struggle with their weight, the more money they make. They want you to be trapped in their world and for you to see them as the solution to your weight problems. That's why nobody in the industry is telling you the truth or showing you how simple weight loss is. If they did, the weight loss industry wouldn't make any cash.

They want you to put them on a pedestal and see them as your saviour. They do this by working on short-term weight loss. You lose weight over a short period, tell the world how fantastic their method or product is, they get more paying customers, and you gain the weight back on. They win, and you lose. They're getting free advertising and more money; you're left scratching your head. The frustrating thing is that you blame yourself rather than their trickery and return to purchase their method or product to try again, giving them even more of your hard-earned cash.

If the Wild West of the weight loss industry isn't giving you a clear direction, then surely healthcare would? Unfortunately, they're implementing weight loss injections or pills into their arsenal, but that won't work for you either. They're trying to patch you up with a Band-Aid, as that's their job. Covering up the underlying issue and hoping it will fix itself isn't a good solution. Medical students are only taught about ten to twenty-four hours over a five-year degree in nutrition. Our problem is we trust everything a person in a white coat tells us. For most things, that's understandable, but I don't think their lack of nutrition and weight loss lectures provides them with grounds to advise the public on how to be healthy and lose weight correctly.

An injection or pill is not the solution to your weight loss problem. What happens when you stop taking them? Your weight is just going to go back up. A gastric band means you must live a life of restriction and tiny portions for the rest of your life. That doesn't sound very fun, and it's worse than feeling unable to lose weight. Nobody will live a happy life if they can only consume a handful of strawberries for their dinner. How do you think that would affect your mental health? I love and fully support the NHS, but they've got it wrong regarding weight loss. A band-aid solution is only going to make weight loss feel hard.

If healthcare can't provide us with a clear direction, surely government policy would provide us with it? You have a better chance of the cookie-selling girl guides offering sound dietary advice. They don't know their falafel from their fruit. They talk the talk on their website, but I don't think banning the advertising of high-fat, sugar and salt foods on TV and online before 9pm will change much. We aren't educated on how to eat healthily in school. If we're supposed to live an active life, then one hour a week of PE at school won't cut it. If we are supposed to exercise at least twice per week, surely this should be the minimum requirement for PE in schools. How do you think your weight and eating habits would be if you were educated on how to live a healthy life?

Finally, we have the media. They've ruined people's lives, so I don't think they're to be trusted. They spit out poor articles to provide content to their readers. Their sole objective is to get you to click on their article by jumping on trends and gimmicks, not to give you the key information you need. This means they will change the weight loss methods each week, confusing their readers. It causes diet hopping each time you read something different. Even if some magazines are trying to help, there is no synchronicity, preventing us from being told the answer to this simple question, "How do I lose weight and keep it off?".

Reason 4 - People resort to extremes when they hear conflicting messages

All this hot air is creating a whirlwind of confusion in your mind. One person says you should cut out carbs; the other says you need to cut out fats and increase your carbs. How can this be? You're stuck as the rope in a game of tug of war. Unfortunately, when we hear conflicting messages, we resort to extremes, such as going Keto, consuming five hundred calories a day, or drinking a disgusting concoction of apple cider vinegar, green tea, and meal replacement sachets. It's these extremes that nobody has to do to lose weight, but when everyone is singing different lyrics to the same song, which words are correct? On the one hand, resorting to extremes makes sense, but on the other, it's excessive. You're fucked before you even begin.

When there is no clear direction and endless conflicting messages, there's only one natural instinct in this scenario: resort to the most extreme. If you're going to set off on your weight loss journey, you want results and feel if any of the various methods will work, then it will be the most extreme. Plus, it sounds pretty challenging, and humans love telling others how hard things are, even if they want things to be easier. You won't be impressed if I told you I walked up a hill, but you'll definitely be impressed with me telling you how I climbed Mount Everest in 2016.

If one person tells you weight loss is pretty straightforward and requires little effort, you won't believe them as it sounds too good to be true. We are programmed to think weight loss requires sacrifice, struggles, and sadness. It's like the world telling us we had too much of a good time when we were gaining weight, so it's punishing us. By resorting to extremes, you're making things harder for yourself. You also won't be able to stick to this new extreme way of living. This false belief is one of the traps the diet world has set out for you. The feeling of needing to resort to extremes to lose weight means you will be reliant on them.

Unfortunately, you probably still don't believe me when I tell you weight loss can easily be achieved. You will do if you keep reading though. Instead of working harder, you need to think smarter. Reading this book is a smart move. It might take you a few hours to read, and you will have to concentrate on the content and think about the actions you need to take. However, this is a smart use of your energy and time, as it will allow you to lose weight smoothly. By the end of this book, you won't have to resort to extremes or be depleted of energy. You will have created a smart strategy to prevent you from resorting to extremes. Then, it will be your turn to tell people how weight loss is straightforward and have them not believe you.

Reason 5 - Restriction allows us to feel a sense of control

Humans love to feel in control and certainly hate being out of it unless it's freshers' week at University. Control provides a feeling that everything will be ok and you will achieve what you want. This control on your weight loss journey is performed through restrictive diets, which I call 'no' diets. These 'no' diets consist of people saying no to things like alcohol, chocolate, bread, sweets, biscuits, and many other things they enjoy, sapping all the enjoyment out of food. Don't get me wrong, healthy food is delicious, but life without a glass of wine on a summer's day or a freshly baked loaf of bread doesn't sound fun to me. At first, you feel in complete control of your eating habits. No means no. There are no grey areas. Everything is either black or white. Yes or no. However, it would be best to think long-term to achieve your weight loss goal. How long can you not have your favourite foods? What do you think will happen when you eventually have them again?

One thing you can't do is have control through force. Restriction may make weight loss easy for a week or two, but at some point, it will backfire. You can't control a horse by whacking it with a stick. It will buck you off and, if it could speak, would tell you to F@@k off too. We restrict ourselves because, a lot of the time, control through restriction is all we have. Reasons one to four create this. How does restriction make you feel? How many times have you tried to lose weight in the past through restriction and sacrifice, only to find that all that effort gets nothing in return? How long did you keep it off if you achieved some form of weight loss? At some point, did you lose control?

Restricting ourselves from certain foods, activities, or behaviours segregates us from others. And remember, humans love to be a part of something and prefer being in tribes. Segregation is just going to lead to sadness. Sadness isn't going to lead to success. Long-term control is achieved in a relaxed and casual manner. Think of Roger Federer playing tennis or Lionel Messi playing football. Whilst everyone else is frantically running around, they're graceful. Those who rush around and force things are the ones who lose. I need you to have control of your weight in a relaxed and casual manner, so you win. That's what winners do. They make it look like they're not even trying. Be laissez-faire and allow things to take care of themselves. Patience is not simply the ability to wait but how we behave while waiting. No matter what you try to do, you cannot force the desired endpoint. The best of anything cannot be rushed.

Reason 6 - Being too hard on yourself makes weight loss feel hard

"I'm fat", "I can't do this", "I'm a failure", "I can't stick to a diet". These are the inner thoughts people have about themselves. Each one is a negative perception of their body, personality, or behaviours, and breaking out of this thought pattern can be difficult, making weight loss hard.

WHY WEIGHT LOSS IS HARD

You may not realise it, but these inner thoughts have created a glass ceiling - an invisible barrier that limits who you can be and what you can achieve. You can see the light but must break the glass to achieve your weight loss goal. It's not weight loss that's hard; it's breaking the glass and setting yourself free.

Being too hard on yourself fixes the glass ceiling in place, preventing you from pursuing things that give you a happy heart and a sense of achievement. The punishment and pain you place doesn't gain anything other than frustration. This harsh treatment of the mind and body comes from the critic within, filling you with self-doubt and creating limited thinking. The inner critic causes you to filter life through a lens of misperception. Instead of thinking about what is possible, you spend time thinking about what isn't. Your inner critic has you striving for perfection when we all know this isn't attainable for anybody. It encourages you to believe that good isn't great and great isn't good enough. This then sets the chain of events where you're being too hard on yourself because you're striving for perfection, forcing yourself to try harder and sacrifice more. All of this leads to feelings of negativity, which feeds your inner critic and fuels the fire of negative emotions.

What happens is this barrage of negativity strengthens your inner critic. It breeds more thoughts like 'Why would you want to lose weight when you aren't able to do it?', 'Why do you think you deserve happiness with a new body you love?' and 'Why do you think you can get in shape when the world is more obese now than ever before?' When you consciously or subconsciously absorb even the smallest nugget of negativity, it slowly chips away at your confidence. It causes you to stay exactly where you are rather than motivating you to begin moving forward. One of the most obvious implications of the inner critic is that it tells you it's protecting you and helping you strive for more, but that's far from the truth.

As we've already identified, it's whacked a glass ceiling above you that needs to be shattered. Where's Miley Cyrus and her wrecking ball when you need it? What the inner critic has done is cause greater procrastination, preventing you from moving forward with ease, rendering motivation as your expectations are so high that you're constantly underachieving in your mind. This leads to lower self-control, taking you further from achieving your weight loss goal.

To get rid of your inner critic, you must first take the pressure off and stop being so hard on yourself. This will require consistent attention and practice as you're programmed to be this way due to the five reasons I've already covered in this chapter. It's time to break the chain and smash the glass ceiling. I want you to begin calling out your inner critic when you hear it chirping up. The way to do this is to give it a silly name and start thinking of your inner critic as its own entity. This way, it becomes less threatening as you've disconnected these views from your own. Throw a few expletives or tell it how ridiculous it's been each time you hear it getting louder. It's crazy how good you feel once you've put it in its place. Don't allow the inner critic to speak for you.

WHY WEIGHT LOSS IS HARD

You're not fat; you have body fat to lose. You can lose weight as you're a strong individual. Nobody is calling you a failure, so don't call yourself one. You can't stick to a diet because it's a way of being too hard on yourself. Don't feed the inner critic. Think of the positive things about yourself, both inside and out. Take the pressure off, praise yourself, enjoy the journey, take the correct steps, and celebrate the wins. As the positive feelings continue, you will feel happier, make better decisions and easily achieve your weight loss goal. What words would you use to describe yourself? Are the things you think positive or negative? Are you too hard on yourself? Have you allowed the inner critic to sneak in? How could you prevent the inner critic from taking over?

Reason 7 - Dieting is messing with the body and mind

You know what you want, but have you ever stopped and thought about what your emotions want? All of these restrictions, negative thoughts, and extremities can lead us to have disordered eating and suffer with our mental health. Disordered eating sits between normal eating and an eating disorder, and it's such a common condition that everyone denies they have. This tends to be due to society considering the symptoms as normal and healthy behaviours. These behaviours are even promoted as healthy ways to lose weight, such as fasting, skipping meals, cutting calorie intake to extremely low levels, avoiding a type of food or food group, taking diet pills or having injections. Other symptoms include binge eating,

WHY WEIGHT LOSS IS HARD

self-induced vomiting, or laxative and diuretic misuse. Dieting is one of the most common forms of disordered eating, and it messes with your body and mind.

An eating disorder is not a lifestyle choice; they are severe and damaging to your health. Unfortunately, the diet culture has rewritten the rulebook to make disordered eating appear to be a lifestyle choice and healthy. You need to understand that disordered eating and dieting are among the most common risk factors for developing an eating disorder. They also aren't a healthy way to lose weight, and in the long run, can be highly damaging to your body. Restricting the amount of food you eat to tiny quantities and minimal calories can be dangerous. When the body is starved of food, it responds by reducing the rate at which it burns energy. This means your metabolism slows down, making weight loss difficult in the long run. It also means that your vital organs, such as your brain, heart, lungs, liver and kidneys, function at much lower rates due to being starved of energy. This means they don't function properly, which can lead to illness and disease. A lot of this damage is also irreversible.

Your body is a truly fantastic thing. It runs without you even having to think about the functions and actions it takes. Its sole role is to keep you alive and well. When you drop your food intake too low, it releases a hunger hormone that tells you to eat. Usually, this is a good thing, but not when trying to overrule your body through dieting. You and your body are fighting one another. You want to lose weight, and your body wants to keep what it already has. This is why when you go on a diet, you often find yourself overeating or even binge eating. Feelings of guilt and failure arise from 'falling off the wagon' and being unable to stick to the diet. But it's not your fault. You're not a failure. Your body is trying to look after you.

If your inner critic is the bad guy, your body's hunger hormone is Granny Smith. She's just trying to look after you. "Here, dear, have some more dinner; after seconds, I've got apple pie and custard.". She hasn't got a bad thing to say about you; she wants you to have a full belly and a warm heart. When you restrict your food intake, your body responds by increasing your appetite, so you eat more, which is bad when losing weight. Your body also feels irritable or what's known as hangry these days. Energy levels are low, and the diet rules are broken. Due to your body wanting and needing more energy through food, you binge and overeat. Your body only asks for a couple hundred calories to replenish its stores, but once Granny Smith kicks in, she won't stop feeding you. At a time when your body needs anything, it will always take much more than it needs. You may feel like you've failed, and you've only got yourself to blame due to a lack of motivation and willpower, but it's the structure of a diet's fault, causing Granny Smith to feed you up.

You can't override your body's natural responses. What you can do is plan ahead to prevent them from kicking in. To do this, you must feed your body sufficiently so your hunger hormones don't kick in. This means planning your meals, consuming the required nutrients, and getting sufficient calories. This way, if Granny Smith comes knocking with a banoffee pie, you can say, "No thanks, Granny, I've already eaten." and stay on track. As most people aren't doing this, they are often led back to the diet cycle of restriction with an "I'll do better this time" mindset, and the diet cycle, which destroys your dreams, ambitions, and feelings, fails you again. This is why you think weight loss is hard. Instead, you must focus on treating your body with respect and give it what it needs to prevent disordered eating from kicking in. Don't allow dieting to mess up your body and mind.

Reason 8 - You haven't got a plan

When I say the word plan, what do you think of? Do you think of one of those fancy PDF documents with your workout and diet plan on it? What about one of those on-trend diets? It could be a basic plan such as "I'm going to start exercising and control my eating habits". All may sound like plans, but they're far from it. You don't need a graphic designer; you need expertise. You don't need someone to tell you what to do; you need someone to help you decide the best way for you. You don't need a trend; you need something that works. A basic plan is a statement. What we believe is the solution to our weight loss problem is merely just something fancy and sellable. Something you think is a plan is nothing short of a piece of paper.

People will find it hard work when they set off to lose weight without a true and personal plan. At times, they will go through the motions, feeling lost, confused, and frustrated. The plan won't feel like their plan. Over time, they will begin to think they don't want to eat certain things on the plan or train a certain way. It will feel like they're following somebody else's way of losing weight because they are. They were inspired by somebody else and encouraged to follow their way. Yet, somebody else's way should never be your way. Although everyone wants the same thing, not everyone likes the same food, has the same lifestyle, or the same personality. This is why only you can create your weight loss plan as you know the most about yourself. Any other plan created by any other person is inferior and redundant.

Pablo Picasso knew that inspiration was only a tiny part of any effort. The creative process is one of planning, failing and planning anew. But those plans are rooted in a belief that they will work. Without that faith, no plan will clear the hurdles that block the progress of any project. For you to believe in your plan, you must create it. In doing so, you become a creator, just like Pablo himself. You create a plan that will deliver a masterpiece. The process will flow, the confidence will grow, and you will soon see how a plan you create makes weight loss easier.

A successful plan takes a holistic approach. You must understand many parts of your life must be implemented into your plan. It's not solely about what you will eat and how you will exercise. You must implement the way you think, feel, and the environment you are in. How will you act throughout your journey, make the necessary changes, and overcome any obstacles along the way?

WHY WEIGHT LOSS IS HARD

Most importantly, how will you feel throughout your journey? Your head and heart must work together in an environment that allows you to thrive. When you take a holistic approach, your plan will be easier to follow.

Reason 9 - It's not you, it's the situation you're in

For anything to change, someone has to start acting differently. Although they have to alter parts of their lifestyle, it's not them as a person that's the problem; it's the person's situation. A person and a person's situation may sound similar; however, they are two different things. Suppose you feel overwhelmed about losing weight because of a lack of time, distractions, procrastination, or the wide range of information out there. In that case, you believe it's you who is the problem. You try things and fail, so you are at fault, assuming you've only got yourself to blame. It's easy to blame yourself, but it's not you that's failing; it's the situation or system failing you. We tend to blame ourselves rather than look at how our surroundings and situations encourage us to behave in a certain way.

Let me tell you the story of a woman named Amanda who wanted to lose weight. She travelled a lot due to her job and had a pile of work waiting for her when she got home. She wanted to lose weight by cooking healthy meals and exercising, so she decided to join the gym. Amanda felt that if she joined a gym, she would go and managed to do so for a couple of weeks. The more she went to the gym, the higher the pile of work got, and the less time she had to cook healthy meals. Although

WHY WEIGHT LOSS IS HARD

Amanda regularly attended the gym, she didn't lose weight. She was stressed with all the work she had to do, which led to her grabbing some dinner and chocolate after the gym. This prevented her from losing weight because she ate more than she was burning off at the gym. Once she eventually sat down to make a dent in the pile of work, she would open the chocolates and graze whilst responding to emails. When the chocolates were gone and the laptop shut, she would grab a glass of wine to switch off to get to sleep.

Although Amanda tried hard to lose weight, it wasn't going to happen for her. She was growing frustrated with herself and could feel herself tensing up. Negative thoughts about herself crept into her mind. The inner critic took to the stage with renditions of "I'm a Failure", "I Can't Do This", and the best seller "I'm Destined to be This Way for the Rest of My Life". Losing weight felt hard to achieve. No matter how much she tried, it was never going to happen. She was stuck between a rock and a hard place. Is Amanda a failure? Is it her fault? Or is the situation preventing her from achieving her goal?

When you've unsuccessfully tried to lose weight in the past, it was almost certainly because of your situation at the time. You were probably just like Amanda, who was great at trying but had a situation problem. When you failed to lose weight, did you blame yourself too? Amanda had plenty of positive traits. She didn't need to change herself; she needed to open her eyes to see her situation. Many parts of her situation could change with minimal effort to allow her to lose weight. She could communicate with colleagues and reduce her workload by delegating at work rather than trying to do everything herself. She could organise her weekly meals and make most of them at the weekend when she has more time. She could claim back over one hour of her evening if she did shorter exercise sessions at home instead of going to the gym. If she made these changes to her situation, there would be much less resistance fighting her. Communication, organisation, and realising there are only so many hours in each day have altered her situation. These changes give her more time, allowing her to eat better and be more consistent with her exercise sessions. Once she changes her situation, she will feel it's possible to lose weight as her week will be clearer, and she will feel happier. How can you make your situation more manageable to allow you to lose weight?

We tend to attribute people's behaviour to their core character rather than their situation. This is known in psychology as the fundamental attribution error. We don't know why somebody is unable to lose weight in the same way we don't know why somebody is speeding down the motorway. When you stop to think about why somebody is doing something, you will help balance out your perspective. This will prevent you from looking through the lens of a single negative quality and instead see them as a person stuck in a bad situation. Amanda is driven and successful, yet her situation never allowed her to feel it or others to see it. This brings us to the final reason why you think weight loss is hard.

Reason 10 - You're exhausted trying to lose weight

We're all expected to work harder, be more productive, and achieve many things. Life is shouting at us to get up and do more. People on the internet show how much they get done in a day. Friends patronise you as they constantly tell you to do more. They always have time to go to the gym, so should you! "Sling it Karen with your free time, no stress, and live-in nanny" runs through your head. She doesn't know what a good days graft looks like. Deep down, you know why you can't do what she can do; you've got a lot on your plate at the moment. Yet, at the same time, you still have a sense of guilt, laziness, and inferiority. People on the internet are better than you. Friends around you are better than you. Life is shouting at you to get up and do more; piss right off. Comparison syndrome is the bane of my life. We are all in different situations. It's time for it to do one.

Have you ever been called lazy by someone? I bet you've thought that other people believed you were lazy, and I bet that hurts. Just like Amanda, you've been in a situation problem which you haven't identified until now. The nine reasons have caused you to feel stuck in a rut. You've been attempting to lose weight but failing, taking action but getting nothing back, and thinking negatively of yourself for these reasons. All this can lead you to think, "What's the point?". Your mood is deflated, and your energy levels are exhausted, but the thought of giving up isn't because you're lazy. You've been trying, and you've been trying so hard. You've attempted ten ways to lose weight, with everyone being unsuccessful. Each time has knocked some energy out of you until you feel you've gone ten rounds with Tyson Fury. Weight loss is hard because you've worn yourself out so much you've become burnt out. Even when you feel like you're trying, you're too exhausted to continue or even begin.

When we are exhausted, we suddenly stop trying to lose weight. You don't consciously make this decision; your body does. The mind is exhausted due to the stress, the pressure, and the fear of failure. The body is depleted due to poor diets, vigorous exercises and low calories. The body throws in the towel at the end of the tenth round, knowing it can't continue. After your concerted effort, you need some time to recover. Sometimes, it's only a couple of weeks; others, it's several years. It all depends on how exhausted you've been from trying in the past and what other things you have going on in your life. These are when your inner critic begins to laugh at you and tell you you're a failure. These are the times when you feel others judge you each time you eat or sit on the sofa. You're exhausted, and the only way to successfully lose weight is when you're re-energised and have found a way of losing weight that doesn't feel like a fight with a heavyweight boxer.

This period is a time to recover, rest, switch off, and do things you enjoy doing. For some, it's going for walks in the countryside. For others, it's catching up with friends for a few drinks. You see, once you've had a period of exhaustion and burnout, you need time to overcome the fatigue. You may feel like you're not doing anything, but you are. There's an upside to this downtime, and you will benefit from it in the long run. Everything begins with a feeling and your weight loss journey is no different. You will be ready to lose weight when you feel happier, less stressed, and more energised. Until that time, you're best not trying. When you have positive feelings, you will take positive actions. When you take positive actions, you will get positive results. When you feel like the world is shouting at you to get up and go, wait. Only take action when you feel energised and ready to go.

Do you see why you've been thinking weight loss is hard?

The ten reasons are intertwined. It's not one thing making weight loss hard, so putting your finger on what's preventing you from losing weight can be challenging. When you've wondered why weight loss is hard, you've probably never thought it was due to a variety of reasons that are bigger than a lack of willpower or a love of carbs. It's who you listen to, what you know, how you act, and how you feel. Now you know why you've felt stuck, you can take the shackles off and be free. You can explore a way of losing weight that's been standing right in front of you for all these years. A method that isn't reinventing the wheel; it's just using the wheels how they should be used. It makes sense to keep the wheels circular instead of making them square.

You must no longer listen to the noise around you to make weight loss easy. Just because people are shouting the loudest, it doesn't make them right. Instead, you will listen to yourself, as you know best. You know the most about yourself, so you must listen to what your body and mind are saying. You will no longer mirror other people's actions as you will no longer feel lost or insecure. Instead, you will mirror your own positive actions by discovering what you're already doing well and cloning them. This will increase self-confidence and create an inner strength to allow you to be the best version of yourself.

Suppose you no longer listen to the noise around you and only mirror your own positive actions. In that case, you will no longer have to resort to extremes as you won't hear conflicting messages. This book provides the information you need to succeed on your weight loss journey. There's no mumbo jumbo in this book, so you won't make the mistake of resorting to extremes. It's my job to keep things simple and clear. You will know what I ask of you and what you need to do. You will realise you don't have to restrict yourself to feel a sense of control. I encourage you to eat, not diet. To live your life, not live in fear. You will be in control of your weight loss journey due to the message being simple.

If being too hard on yourself makes weight loss hard, what do you think being kind to yourself will do? Forcing yourself to do things and thinking negatively of yourself isn't going to get you anywhere. When something feels hard, it is hard. When something feels easy, it is easy. Everything begins with a feeling, so you must feel good, be positive, and take it easy on yourself. If you praise yourself, weight loss will be more effortless. If you understand that failure is a way to learn, weight loss will be stress-free. If you decide to be kind, weight loss will be a walk in the park.

The dieting world has been failing you and keeping you as one of its prisoners. Put your middle finger up to the dieting world and tell it to swivel. For too long, diets have messed with your body and mind. Weight loss will be easy if you don't listen to them anymore. If you're to take inspiration from a particular tribe, ensure it's the healthy weighted people. I will show you a way of eating that will work for you. This way of eating will give your body plenty of energy. You will feel satisfied with the quantities of your meals and relaxed knowing how to eat well and plan your meals accordingly.

This book aims to help you create a weight loss roadmap. This is a plan on steroids. Everything you need to factor into your plan is included in this book. If this sounds overwhelming, then remember it's a simple step-by-step process. You won't even notice all the parts of the plan, but they will come together to guarantee success. You will get excited as the more you move through the book, the more real achieving your weight loss goal will be. Your roadmap will factor in the situation you are in as a successful plan must consider a person's environment. You will be encouraged to think about your situation to ensure no obstacles or challenges get in your way.

Being exhausted trying to lose weight, makes weight loss hard and unachievable. This is the final time you will have to attempt to lose weight. You've trusted me to deliver, and that's exactly what I will do. I don't wish you to spend exhaustible energy and time creating a weight loss roadmap that won't work. It would be best if you weren't exhausted while on your weight loss journey. I know energy is exhaustible, so I ask you to do one thing at a time. Focus on the content and actions of one chapter before you move on to the next. You can take your time with this book. Rome wasn't built in a day; neither is your weight loss roadmap. One thing the Romans were good at once they got going was building straight roads, and you will build one that takes you directly to your destination. Instead of exhaustion, I will energise you both physically and mentally.

Your weight loss journey is not a sprint. You've just been programmed to believe it is. Yes, Usain Bolt has all the fame, but you must be Eliud Kipchoge. If you're left thinking, who's that? He's the only person to run the marathon in under two hours at 1:59:40. That should be your goal: to run the fastest marathon you can run. To run this crazy time, Kipchoge was joined by forty-one pacemakers who rotated twice each lap and ran in a V-formation to ensure Kipchoge could run the fastest time possible with the least amount of energy. This shape helped the runners make better progress. The front runner breaks up the wall of air the athletes run into, leaving a wake of swirling air behind, helping to reduce resistance to the runner's further back. Kipchoge was placed at the bottom of the formation with two pacemakers running behind him.

That's not the only thing that aided Kipchoge in breaking the two-hour marathon barrier. Pacing lasers guided the pacemakers and the leading runner, allowing them to run at a precise pace to ensure energy was not lost in unwanted acceleration. The route was carefully chosen to ensure no effort was wasted on battling the wind or any directional or incline changes. This was achieved because most of the course was lined with tall trees, reducing wind further, and the course was very flat. The location of the race was chosen because its time zone was close to that of Kaptagat, Kenya, where Kipchoge trains. This meant Kipchoge would not be affected by jet lag or have his sleeping and eating patterns disrupted. The route was picked to be at a low altitude to increase oxygen in the air and thus improve performance. Kipchoge wore an improved version of Nike's previously unreleased Vaporfly Next% running shoes, which claimed to improve running economy by four percent. His shoes had a carbon-fibre plate fitted in their chunky foam sole, which helped propel him forward. Hydration was provided by a team coordinator on a bicycle and not via the usual water station method to save time.

    All these things may not seem much, but they propelled Kipchoge to achieve something remarkable. You can do something remarkable too. The story of Eluids success shows that an extraordinary achievement isn't achieved by focusing on one thing. It's a combination of all things that come together and allow you to achieve a big goal. You must look at things holistically and search for the marginal gains to streamline your weight loss journey and lead you to the finish line. I'm not telling you to get forty-one people to join you on your weight loss journey, to go out and spend £250 on a fancy pair of trainers, or to get your partner to keep providing you with drinks. It's almost time for you to begin creating the plan that's going to help you run your marathon in the quickest time possible. Slowly factor in all the things that will allow you to glide to the finish line with as little effort as possible. It's your time to shine, your time to break your weight loss record and your time to do things your way. Like those pacemakers, I will be with you every step of the way, guiding you, motivating you, and making your journey as easy as possible. Are you ready? Let's do this.

2

UNDERSTANDING BODYWEIGHT

Before I help you lose weight, I must inform you how your body works. Only then will you take the correct actions. People tell you what to do without telling you why you should do it. "Here's your diet plan and exercises" isn't enough. They must tell you the reasons behind the plan, diet, or exercise routine. They need to inform you how weight loss works. This chapter helps you understand body weight. My first question is, what do you know about body weight? Do you believe all weight loss is the same? What is your body weight made up of? How do you lose weight? Where does fat loss go? How much weight can you lose each week? Take a minute to decide if you know the answers to these questions. If you do, what are your answers?

Body weight is complex. Many cogs within the body play a role in body weight regulation, making it a confusing and contradicting topic. As I mentioned in Chapter Two, people resort to extremes when they hear conflicting messages. This is why people try to eat five hundred calories a day, only eat one food or food group, do two hours of exercise daily to lose weight, or follow a ketogenic diet. Any person who is a competent weight loss coach should be able to explain body weight simply so it's easy for all to understand. I guess the pressure is on me in this chapter.

Let's begin with a person's body mass index, which is abbreviated to BMI. This is a person's weight in kilograms divided by the squared height in metres. A healthy BMI is between 18.5 and 25.0. Falling within this range is a great weight loss target. Instead of working out your own, use a BMI calculator online. It will show your current BMI score, along with your healthy BMI weight range. I've provided the categories below.

Below 18.5 – You're in the underweight range
Between 18.5 and 24.9 – You're in the healthy weight range
Between 25 and 29.9 – You're in the overweight range
30 or over – You're in the obese range

Your BMI gives you an idea of how healthy your weight is for your height, which is why it's an excellent place to start. The negative is that it doesn't take into consideration what your body weight is made up of. This is known as your body composition. With a healthy BMI, 25% of a person's weight is comprised of organ weight. That's your brain,

UNDERSTANDING BODYWEIGHT

heart, lungs, liver, kidneys, digestive system, etc. The weight of their bones makes up 12 to 15% of their total body weight. There are approximately 206 bones in the human body that need to be dense and strong to avoid injuries and support us. We are programmed to hate our body fat; however, 3% of a healthy male's body weight and 12% of a healthy female's body weight is made up of essential fat. This is found in muscles, nerve cells, bone marrow, intestines, heart, liver, and lungs and is the fat needed to maintain normal physiological functions. All the types of weight mentioned so far equate to 43-49% of a healthy person's total body weight. Almost 50% of a person's body weight is pretty significant to keep hold of, which is why all types of body weight shouldn't be treated as equal.

When people talk about body weight, they tend to refer to more variable types. Yet, these shouldn't be treated equally either. Another important part of your body composition is your muscle mass, which varies depending on lifestyle, age, and gender. Muscles, attached to bones or internal organs and blood vessels, are responsible for movement. Nearly all movement in the body is the result of muscle contraction. Muscles are also the tissue that makes you look good. When people say they want to tone up, they're referring to having more muscle and less body fat. It requires a lot of energy in the form of calories to function, which means the more muscle you have, the more you can eat without gaining weight. An increase in lean muscle mass leads to greater control of your body weight. It's a good idea to keep hold of the muscle mass

UNDERSTANDING BODYWEIGHT

you have and, if possible, increase the amount of muscle you have too.

Earlier, I spoke about essential fats and the importance of keeping hold of this weight. There is also a classification of your body composition called non-essential fat. A healthy person's non-essential body fat percentage would be approximately 12% for men and 15% for women. As it's non-essential, it will vary from person to person. Generally, a healthy male's total body fat percentage would be between 10 and 23%, depending on age. A healthy female's total body fat percentage would be between 16 and 28%. This percentage is for both essential and non-essential body fats as a total. It can be challenging to accurately gauge a person's total body fat percentage; however, scales that measure body fat and muscle mass percentages provide a rough idea. Out of all of the types of body composition mentioned so far, non-essential fat is the only weight you should aim to lose. This is why weight loss professionals refer to weight loss as fat loss.

By now, you understand that the only weight you should lose is non-essential body fat. One more thing that affects your total body weight is water. This is because your body comprises 50 to 70% water. Your bones, muscles and organs all contain water. Your body is a massive sponge. The easiest way to drop weight quickly is to squeeze the sponge and decrease the amount of water in the body. However, all this will do is make you feel good for one second when you step on the scales due to having the same body composition as a rice cake.

UNDERSTANDING BODYWEIGHT

Carbohydrates love water, soaking it up and retaining it in the body. If you take out carbohydrates from your diet, your water levels decrease in the body, leading to temporary weight loss. This is how no or low-carbohydrate diets trick you into believing you've lost fat weight when all you've done is lose water weight. Think of a plant without water; the pot might be lighter, but it looks and feels awful. It's better to remain hydrated and look like a perky plant that's flourishing. Even if this means you're a little heavier.

Due to 50-70% of your body consisting of water, you must understand that water weight causes your weight to fluctuate by up to six pounds per day naturally. This weight fluctuation depends on how hydrated you are, what foods you've eaten, and your hormones. For this reason, it's best to weigh yourself first thing in the morning after you've been to the loo. It's also essential to make sure that you look at your average weigh-ins rather than what it says when you step on the scales once. Always take the average of four weigh-ins to calculate your accurate body weight.

We are often influenced to lose as much weight, as quickly as possible, which can lead people away from only trying to lose body fat. Your weight drops quicker when losing muscle and fat simultaneously. This is because muscle weight is made up of around 75% water, whereas fat is made up of approximately 10% water. Watching the pounds fly off might feel good initially, but it won't leave you feeling amazing when you achieve your weight loss goal. You won't look great as you will have lost lots of muscle mass, making your body look like a deflated

UNDERSTANDING BODYWEIGHT

balloon. Muscle is what makes you look toned and feel strong. Losing muscle also makes controlling your body weight more difficult, meaning the lost weight will be regained at some point, as muscle plays a vital role in body weight regulation.

The way to ensure you only lose body fat is to take things a little slower than others. A healthy amount of fat loss is 1-2 pounds per week. Anything over this number will always be water or muscle weight for most people. Instead of crash dieting, place yourself in a calorie deficit of five hundred calories and consume sufficient protein to maintain your muscle mass. This is something I will cover in a later chapter. Weight loss should always be fat loss. In this book, I will refer to fat loss as weight loss, as this is the term you would use. My objective is to speak in your vocabulary. The next step is to understand how weight loss and weight gain happen.

Weight loss occurs when you consume fewer calories than your body burns off. Calories are units of energy that we get from food and burn off through living and activity. You can lose weight by reducing your calorie intake to reduce calorie input or increasing your activity levels to increase your calorie output, creating a calorie deficit. Weight gain occurs when you consume more calories than your body burns, creating a calorie surplus. Each time you're in a calorie surplus, your body will store excess calories as body fat. Each time you're in a calorie deficit, your body will use the stored body fat as energy for the body, leading to fat loss.

UNDERSTANDING BODYWEIGHT

Consuming fewer calories than your body burns off is how all weight loss methods work. This is how your body loses weight. It doesn't lose weight because it doesn't have carbohydrates, that's water weight. It doesn't work through syns, points, diets, or fasting; they're all tactics. Diets and weight loss methods are all packaged in different ways. Yet, they have the same formula: being in a calorie deficit. Each tactic or tool wants to stand out from the crowd, sound unique, and grab everyone's attention, so you're attracted to follow them over all other potential weight-loss approaches. Think about the first reason why I said weight loss is hard, 'He who shouts the loudest gets heard (unfortunately)'. The packaging conceals the formula of being in a calorie deficit to lose weight because it wants to be different. This, in turn, causes people to believe that being in a calorie deficit is a weight loss method when it's actually how you lose weight.

Do you drive a Ford Fiesta, an Audi A4, or a Porsche 911? It doesn't matter, as they all work in the same way. You turn the engine on, put your foot down on the accelerator, the wheels get moving, and you hit the brakes so you don't crash into another car. They look different and have varied features, but how a vehicle works and the purpose of driving are the same. The wheels move, getting you from where you are to where you want to be. Diets work the same way. They're simply vehicles to your destination. Vehicles have different badges, different types of people who drive them, and different features; in the same way, diets have different labels, sound different and have different kinds of people following them. A car is a car, and a diet is a diet. All cars work the same. All diets work the same. Calories in versus calories out is the fundamental concept of body weight regulation, and it's as close to scientific fact as we can get. Instead of talking horsepower and cup holders in the car park, get in the car and drive to your destination. Instead of debating what diet to follow, put yourself in a calorie deficit, and you will reach your destination.

The calories in part is straightforward. It is simply the food and drink you consume. You control and assess your calorie intake by looking at how many calories are in the foods and drinks you're consuming. When assessing the calories out part of the equation, many different parts come together to create your total daily calorie expenditure. This is the total amount of calories you burn each day. I will cover the actual amount later on.

You must first understand that Exercise Activity Thermogenesis (EAT) is responsible for only around 5% of a healthy adult's total daily calorie expenditure. These are the calories you burn off when exercising. If they're only responsible for such a tiny amount, why does everyone feel they need to exercise to lose weight? The reason is that although exercise is only responsible for 5% of total calorie burn, it can be increased, as it's a variable part of your total calorie expenditure. If you're not exercising, your EAT totals 0% of your total calorie burn. You have control over how many calories you burn off through exercise, like you have control over how many calories you consume.

UNDERSTANDING BODYWEIGHT

Non-Exercise Activity Thermogenesis (NEAT) is the calories you burn when doing various activities that aren't exercise. This includes walking, cooking, fidgeting, playing with the kids, doing household chores, sitting down, and carrying things. All movements come under the category of activity. Calories burnt through activity equate to 15% of a healthy adult's daily calorie burn. Once again, the amount of calories you burn through activity is variable, allowing you to increase this amount and burn even more calories daily. If you don't wish to drop your calorie intake through food down too low, you can place yourself in a calorie deficit by increasing your EAT and NEAT. If you aren't currently active, your NEAT could be much lower than 15%, and losing weight would be much easier if you were more active.

The Thermic Effect of Food (TEF) relates to the energy required to digest, absorb and store food and is responsible for 10% of a healthy adult's daily calorie burn. In short, eating food burns calories. If your diet isn't great, your TEF will be lower than it should be, meaning you burn fewer calories each day, making weight loss more difficult. The simple solution is consuming a range of whole foods that cause the body to work harder to digest, absorb, and store. This is an area I will cover in greater detail later on in this book. The energy required to digest each macronutrient (Fats, Carbs, Proteins) can be expressed as a percentage of the energy provided by the food group. Fat provides nine calories per gram; its TEF is 0-3%. Carbohydrate provides four calories per gram; its TEF is 5-10%. Protein provides four calories per gram; its TEF is

UNDERSTANDING BODYWEIGHT

20-30%. More energy is required to break down protein as it takes longer to be digested. This is why protein makes you feel fuller for longer. Processed foods are already broken down, making it easier for your body to digest, absorb, and store. To ensure your TEF is 10%, consume whole foods and ensure you consume sufficient protein.

Your Basal Metabolic Rate (BMR) accounts for 70% of a healthy person's daily calorie burn. This is how many calories your body burns at rest. You burn 600-800 calories while you're asleep. Sounds pretty good, doesn't it? Although your body is lying down and resting, many things are happening behind the scenes. It performs basic yet essential functions to sustain life. This includes the vital roles of breathing, circulating blood around the body, processing nutrients, regenerating cells throughout the body, brain and nerve functions, controlling body temperature, and contracting muscles. Your BMR varies by gender, age, ethnicity, height, weight, and body composition. The more you weigh, the higher your BMR. The energy cost of weight-bearing activities such as walking and standing is related to body weight. It is, therefore, higher the heavier you are. As you lose weight, your BMR will reduce due to a decrease in the energy cost of weight-bearing activities. From the age of 30, you begin to lose as much as 3-5% muscle mass per decade, meaning a total loss of approximately 30% in your lifetime. This is why losing weight as you get older can feel more difficult, as your total calorie burn reduces the less muscle you have. To combat this and keep your BMR high, do some form of resistance training to maintain or increase your muscle mass. The various ways your body uses and burns calories combine to create your total calorie burn. As a recap, your Exercise Activity Thermogenesis (EAT) can be increased by doing more exercise. Non-Exercise Activity Thermogenesis (NEAT) can be increased by being more active. The Thermic Effect of Food (TEF) can be increased by consuming whole foods and more protein. Your Basal Metabolic Rate (BMR) is responsible for sustaining life, decreases as you lose weight and age, and increases as you increase your muscle mass by doing some form of resistance training. These are the key parts to remember about your total calorie burn. I have used some big words in this section. I won't be using them again, as I wish for you to understand what I'm talking about.

In the rest of the book, I will refer to each complicated word as the following.

Exercise Activity Thermogenesis = Exercise
Non-Exercise Activity Thermogenesis = Activity
Thermic Effect of Food = Balanced Diet
Basal Metabolic Rate = Metabolism

It's time to dig deeper into understanding body weight by explaining body regulation. The body can keep a constant internal environment by making regular adjustments as conditions change inside and outside of the body. This is known as homeostasis. The body is brilliant, and we have the joy of living inside it. The first example of this, which should be easy to understand, is being too hot or cold. Our bodies like to be 37 degrees Celsius. If we get too hot, we start to sweat, as this is our body's way of cooling down to its regulated temperature. If we get too cold, we begin to shiver, as this is our body's way of warming up to its regulated temperature. It does this without us even thinking about it. We can get out of the sun to cool down if we get too hot or put a coat on if we get too cold, but our body will always do whatever it takes to get back to 37 degrees Celsius.

The first example of body regulation was one that we can all relate to. I used it to show you how your body regulates itself, and the above is an easy one to understand. Body regulation can affect your body weight; the first example is your blood sugar levels. I'm sure you've heard of insulin and glucose. Well, they work hand in hand. Insulin is a hormone made in your pancreas and allows your body to use glucose as energy. Glucose is the primary type of sugar in the blood and is the body's primary source of energy. If glucose levels remain high, so will the production of insulin. If glucose levels are low, the level of insulin drops and glucose increases. They work hand in hand to regulate your blood sugar levels. When blood sugar levels are low, your body will ask you to take in sugar; this is where the problem starts. All your body needs is less than half a teaspoon to be happy. Instead, we drink a can of Coke or have a Mars bar containing seventy-four teaspoons. Our body is clever in regulating our blood sugar levels. Still, the human error of consuming

UNDERSTANDING BODYWEIGHT

too much sugar creates greater insulin spikes and more calories from the sugar consumed.

Regulation is a wonderful thing, as it's incredible what the body does behind the scenes. Your body likes to ensure you're in a stable environment by having set points. Your temperature regulator will ensure you remain at 37 degrees Celsius, and your blood sugar regulator will ensure your blood sugar levels remain stable. These set points are where your body wants to be, and the same goes for your weight. Your body has a weight set point. This biological control method in humans actively regulates weight towards a predetermined set weight for each individual. A person of a healthy weight doesn't appear to have any weight concerns due to their body's weight regulation. The longer they're at a healthy weight, the easier it is to maintain it. Suppose they have a day where they over-consume calories. In that case, the body will rebalance over the following days by adjusting its energy intake via decreased appetite or increased energy expenditure via greater movement.

This is excellent news for people of a healthy weight, yet it's terrible news for people who wish to lose weight. The body adapts over time and the longer you've been at a certain weight, the more it will believe this is the weight it should be. How long have you been at your current weight? If it has been for a while, this will be your set point. How long has it taken for you to gain this weight? If it has gradually crept up, it will have to gradually creep back down. If you drop weight quickly, your body will want to return to its original weight as soon as possible. In short, your body's role is to keep you alive and to remain in a stable environment. To do this, it wants you to consume food and move less. The next time you find yourself eating or sitting on the sofa instead of exercising, understand this is your body's way of keeping you stable, safe and alive.

If you're left scratching your head, wondering how on earth you'll lose weight when your body is fighting you, don't worry. The reason why I've explained this terrible news is so you understand it's not your fault you've regained weight after previous weight loss attempts. Approximately 80% of people who lose weight gain it all back. This is not a coincidence. It's not due to the individual being lazy or gluttonous. It's due to your body forcing you to take actions that lead your weight back to its set point. I need you to understand your weight set point so you can factor it into your weight loss journey. Your current weight set point isn't always going to be your weight set point. It can vary, and it's my job to help you bring it down.

Earlier, I explained to you how weight loss works. You now understand weight loss is achieved by being in a calorie deficit. You can eat fewer calories or burn more calories to achieve this. I now need to introduce the other players to the minefield of weight loss. The first is the hormone Ghrelin. In chapter two, I spoke about Granny Smith wanting to feed you. Granny Smith is Ghrelin. The hormone in your body that initiates eating and tells you to eat food. When you place yourself in a calorie deficit to try and lose weight, Ghrelin signals a shortage in energetic

UNDERSTANDING BODYWEIGHT

requirements, and the level of Ghrelin in the body increases.

Every action has an equal and opposing reaction, and that's how you maintain set points and regulate things in the body. If you have the hunger hormone Ghrelin telling you when you're hungry and when you need to eat, you must have a hormone telling you when you're full. This hormone is called Leptin. It plays a role in the regulation of your appetite and fat storage. It helps inhibit hunger and regulate energy balance so the body does not trigger hunger responses when it does not need energy. Leptin and Ghrelin work together to control your body weight. Leptin decreases your appetite, and Ghrelin increases it based on your body's needs. You don't have to worry about these two hormones or your set point; everything covered in this book will allow you to lower your weight set point while keeping Ghrelin happy.

How do you gain weight if you have a hormone that tells you to stop eating and regulates energy balance? The short answer is that these body regulators can become damaged or broken and stop working correctly. Considering the body temperature regulator example, somebody with severe hypothermia will experience a hot flush in one final attempt to warm up. Due to this, they begin removing their clothes as they feel hot. This system is broken as it doesn't help to get naked when you're freezing cold. Regarding your blood sugar regulator, you can stop responding well to insulin and can no longer use glucose in your blood for energy to make up for it. Your pancreas creates more insulin, and your blood sugar levels increase over time. This is another example of a regulator breaking down. If these regulators can stop working correctly, the same must happen to your body weight regulators too.

Eating until you're full will stretch out your stomach and increase its capacity over time. This may not sound like much; however, if there is more space in the stomach, it will take a greater volume of food before your fullness hormone Leptin kicks in. This can lead to you feeling hungry more often, and over time, you will gradually increase your weight because Leptin no longer tells you when you're full. It's not just the size of your stomach that plays a part in preventing Leptin from signalling when you're full; it's the types of foods you're consuming too. Many processed foods are high in calories yet low in volume. They provide the body with many unnecessary calories and don't fill up the space in your stomach. Many calories can be consumed before Leptin realises and closes the gates. This is an example of your weight regulator being damaged. Still, it's easily fixed by gradually decreasing your portion sizes, consuming low-calorie, high-volume foods, and decreasing the amount of processed food you consume.

Your weight regulator can also become broken, leading to serious weight gain. Leptin resistance is a condition that affects the signalling of your brain and fat cells. The more weight you gain, the greater the fat cells your body produces to store this excess energy. Fat cells produce Leptin in proportion to their size, meaning people with greater amounts of body fat have very high levels of

UNDERSTANDING BODYWEIGHT

Leptin. What usually happens is that high levels of Leptin send a signal to the brain to say that enough energy is stored; however, Leptin resistance means the brain is less sensitive to this signal or fails to recognise the signal completely. If the signals to the brain aren't working, the body will believe it needs to consume more energy, even though plenty is stored. This leads to overeating, which, over time, can lead to serious weight gain. Once again, I don't wish for you to be concerned about this; I need you to understand how weight gain happens.

You know how weight gain occurs and how weight is lost, however, have you ever wondered the answer to this question: Where does body fat go? When your body takes in less energy than it needs, you're in a calorie deficit, meaning your body must use body fat as energy. When body fat is broken down for energy, the pounds you shed are due to two major byproducts being released - Carbon dioxide and water. The carbon dioxide is exhaled during breathing and the water is removed by sweating and urine. If these products are how fat weight is released, do you think exercising would help if you breathe heavily and sweat during a workout?

I don't know about you, but I'm glad I got through that section. If your head hurts, apologies. I've not gone through all of this information to try to impress you. You need to gain a greater understanding of body weight. This way, you know why things are happening, allowing you to notice them when they do. The body is complex, and weight loss can appear complicated, yet most things I've covered are automated responses going on in the body without you realising. Chapter three is the only science chapter; it's simple to understand from here on out. I wish to finish this chapter with something a little lighter: how much weight can you expect to lose?

This chapter has taught you that fat weight is what you should be aiming to lose. I also informed you a healthy amount of fat loss is 1-2 pounds per week. Anything over this number tends to be water or muscle weight. Losing weight over time will gradually lower your weight set point. There's no point in losing weight for it to come back on. It would help if you thought this is the only time you will lose weight for the rest of your life. The only weight worth losing is the weight you will keep off. If this means it's initially slower than others, so be it. Wait and see what happens further down the line when they bounce back to their initial weight, and you continue losing weight. It's essential to manage expectations when setting off on your weight loss journey. Some people are disappointed with two pounds in a week, but it's a fantastic achievement, especially if you do it week in and week out.

Month One - Eight pounds (Just over half a Stone)
Month Three - Twenty-Four pound (Almost two Stone)
Month Six - Forty-Eight Pound (Three and a half Stone)
Month Twelve - Ninety-Six pound (Seven Stone)

As you can see, anybody would be ecstatic with seven stone in one year. Most people don't wish to lose this amount of weight, making their weight loss journey shorter. We are often caught up with how much weight we

UNDERSTANDING BODYWEIGHT

can lose in the shortest time. After all, that's how diets and magazines sell their products or services. They want to sound like the quickest way for you to lose weight, but that's not the impressive part. What's impressive with weight loss is keeping it off and remaining at your target weight. Weight loss should be like an alcoholic anonymous meeting. They stand up, are proud, and inform others how long they've been sober. People ask how much weight you've lost, but the discussion should be about how long you've kept it off for. You don't ask an alcoholic how many bottles they've stopped drinking. Your goal isn't to lose weight the quickest; it's to lose weight and keep it off.

Your To-Do List

1. Record your starting weight and BMI. Don't worry about what the number says. All that matters is that you begin losing weight from that number. You won't know how much weight you've lost if you don't step on now.
2. Snap a few photos of your starting physique. The images will show your transformation. Take pictures from the front, back, and side of your body. You may need help on this one.
3. Record your starting measurements to track lost inches. Record your waist, hip, chest, and arm measurements.

3

THE ELEPHANT AND THE RIDER

If you're left staring into space, wondering how on earth you are going to lose weight when there are ten reasons why you think weight loss is hard and all that science stuff has made your head hurt, do not worry. To overcome these reasons and make the science stuff simple, we need something to make weight loss easy to achieve. The easiest way to do this is to explain the analogy I will use throughout this book, The Elephant and The Rider. Psychologist Jonathan Haidt first introduced this analogy. He argues that we have two sides of our brain. The emotional side of your brain is the Elephant, and the rational side of your brain is the Rider.

The thought that there are two sides to our brain isn't unique to Jonathan Haidt. Other academics agree with the belief there are two sides we must bear in mind. In Daniel Kahneman's Thinking Fast And Slow, he referred to

THE ELEPHANT AND THE RIDER

System One and System Two. System One is fast, instinctive and emotional; System Two is slower, deliberate, and logical. It's also similar to the work of Professor Steve Peters. In his book, The Chimp Paradox, he states there is the human part of our brain and a chimp. The human part represents our logical thinking and the ability to make considered decisions. The chimp is the irrational and impulsive part of the brain that often dominates behaviour.

The Elephant and The Rider analogy was used in a book I read early in my career, Switch, by Chip and Dan Heath. This analogy and book have stuck with me throughout my career. The Rider is a rational thinker, a planner, and an "It makes sense" decision-maker. The Rider understands that it needs to change. The Rider decides to lose weight. The Rider can see a road in front of them that makes sense to follow. Underneath the Rider is the Elephant. The Elephant provides the power for the journey. However, the Elephant is irrational and driven by emotion and instincts. Have you ever done something you shouldn't have and then had a word with yourself, saying, "I shouldn't have done that?" That's the Elephant taking action and the Rider shouting at it afterwards. The Elephant is the part of you that doesn't want to change. It prefers to stay where it is. When pushed, it can back away and head off in the wrong direction.

When the Rider and the Elephant disagree, you've got a problem. The Elephant's desire for instant gratification completely contradicts the Rider's strengths: the ability to think long-term, plan, and think beyond the moment. What

THE ELEPHANT AND THE RIDER

should you do when the Rider wants to lose weight, and the Elephant doesn't? When the Rider wants the body, it's always dreamed of, but the Elephant wants another chippy tea. Most people force themselves to try and lose weight, dismissing the wants and needs of the Elephant. The Rider can get their way temporarily by pulling the reins of the Elephant hard enough and forcing it in the direction they want to go. At some point, however, the Elephant will have enough of this mistreatment and throw the Rider off its back. The Rider must focus on the Elephant's wants and needs to ensure they can steer it in the right direction without any issues.

When you first decided to lose weight, you probably started with the purest intentions. "I need to lose weight for good health"; "I will go for a run every day"; "I will cut my calories"; "I will stop eating chocolate and bread". These are the thoughts that run through your mind at the start, and the logical Rider creates them. The problem is that none of these statements have factored in the emotional Elephant. All the Elephant hears is the Rider shouting, "Me, Me, Me". The logical part of your brain knows that watching what you eat, healthy eating and more movement play a significant part in a person's health and weight loss. Deep down, it knows what to do and knows it's relatively straightforward. Yet, once the Elephant catches a sniff of what the Rider's intentions are, it goes, "No, I'm not doing that!".

The Rider decides to search for a quick fix, hoping it can control the Elephant for the short time needed to lose weight. "If I hold onto the reins so hard, even if the

THE ELEPHANT AND THE RIDER

Elephant turns into a bucking bronco, I can stay on top". You take a look around the weight loss market, full of people shouting the loudest on their stall. "Drop a dress size in a week", shouts one, "Lose a stone in a month", shouts another. You then move around the corner and onto another row of stalls. "No carbs before marbs", shouts the butcher. "Fat makes you fat!" shouts the baker. You continue walking around the market until you select a faddy quick fix to drop weight as quickly as possible.

The pounds fall off over the first couple of weeks, making the Rider delighted. It's been a struggle to keep hold of the Elephant as it's been rather unhappy during this time. The Rider believes if you're comfortable while riding the Elephant, you're probably doing it wrong. With this false belief, the Rider holds on even tighter as the Elephant becomes more challenging to ride. A few more weeks pass and the Elephant decides enough is enough. It's unhappy, hungry, craves foods the Rider has banned and wants to kick back. At the same time, the Rider has used all their strength to keep control of the Elephant, leaving them exhausted. A month passes, and the Elephant and the Rider have had enough. It's been a tough month, and they can't go any further; their weight loss journey grounds to a halt. The Elephant retreats back to the life it was living, taking the Rider with them.

Diets and strenuous workout plans will often fail because the Rider can't keep the Elephant on the road long enough to reach your weight loss destination. The Rider is small compared to the Elephant, limiting the amount of control they can have. Your emotional thinking

THE ELEPHANT AND THE RIDER

is six times stronger than your logical thinking, meaning the Elephant will always win the game of tug-of-war. Emotions win every single time. When used correctly, this strength can provide a drive to succeed you've never experienced before. The Rider needs to use their strength to think logically and the Elephant's emotions to their advantage. Instead of the resistance the Elephant usually puts up, you will find a happy Elephant makes your weight loss journey easier.

If you want to lose weight and keep it off, you must ensure the Elephant and the Rider work together. Both need to be happy with the road they're about to follow, and there can't be resistance between them. When the Elephant and the Rider move together, your weight loss journey becomes easier and more successful. The way to do this is to create a weight loss roadmap.

Your Weight Loss Roadmap

Decisions are inherent to life. We continuously have to make decisions, whether they're simple and day-to-day or complex decisions that lead to significant change. You have decided what to wear today and have also decided it's time for you to lose weight sustainably. We make so many decisions that few of them are made consciously. Most of our day-to-day decisions are made without us even thinking about them. This is because it is not energetically convenient to think about every decision we make. Your body would rather use the energy it sources from food for essential actions such as keeping you alive.

THE ELEPHANT AND THE RIDER

It doesn't care if you call somebody the wrong name or brush your teeth differently. It does care that you breathe and flush out toxins from the body. We also make so many decisions that our brain cannot store all the information on a conscious level due to the required energy. Think of it as deleting stuff from your laptop or phone before you snap any further photos, receive more emails, or download a new app.

Emotions are considered the basis of all decisions we make. Each one of them goes through our emotional filter. With regard to weight loss, the appearance of your body, and the way you feel, understanding the emotional dynamic is very important due to how emotions influence decision-making. Throughout your weight loss journey, many decisions are going to be made. As most of these decisions will be made through this emotional filter, it's best not to leave them to be made last minute. If you decide what to eat when you're starving, you're going to overeat. If you decide whether to exercise once you get home from work, you're going to choose to kick back on the sofa as you're tired. This is why you must develop a clear strategy to lose weight. A structure to your journey. A roadmap to success. This way, you ensure decisions are made in advance, ensuring both the Elephant and the Rider are happy with them.

Each chapter of this book ensures intrinsic motivation by taking you step by step through a clear strategy to lose weight and keep it off. As you work through the chapters, you will gain competence on the subject of weight loss and what to do to ensure you succeed. When you complete the

THE ELEPHANT AND THE RIDER

actions at the end of each chapter, the Elephant will be motivated as it knows its feelings are being factored in and feels you are progressing. Once you combine this with autonomy in decision-making, the Rider will be motivated as they can decide what to eat, how to be active, and how to manage their time to fit into their lifestyle.

Following a different strategy to lose weight provides you with new ways of acting under a range of possibilities and situations during your weight loss journey and throughout your life. This might initially sound scary to both the Elephant and the Rider. They're both scared of the unknown, yet each chapter creates a known route to follow. Creating a new structure by creating your weight loss roadmap allows you to maintain or adapt your current actions rather than flipping your life upside-down. The fear of failure, panic due to lack of planning, and uneasiness of the unknown will not occur as you will have the confidence to do what you consider necessary at the time. This empowers both the Elephant and the Rider, creating a bond between them and a life they're both happy to live. This is achieved by following a roadmap you've created.

It's important to reflect on the existing relationship between you, your weight, and your food intake. You are exposed to different changing scenarios and encouraged to be creative and expressive, allowing you to decide what to do in a particular scenario. Each scenario is an opportunity to learn and develop sequences to determine what works for you, what doesn't, and what you could do differently next time. You look at things more holistically, allowing you to recognise hidden patterns and behaviours between disconnected situations and actions.

By working through this book, you open your mind to new possibilities and solutions. The new knowledge you acquire allows you to self-organise in light of the uncertainty and variability you are exposed to and generate new ways of solving situations. Once again, this isn't scary; it's empowering. When you make the decisions, solve your own problems, and create more and more strategies to overcome any issues, you create change that sticks and weight loss that stays off.

The roadmap you will create throughout this book educates and trains your unconscious decision-making, forming new habits that will become automated over time. Before you know it, you will live a healthy life on autopilot. When this happens, you no longer have to think about your weight. All the stresses and worries you've had in the past disappear. You don't feel like a prisoner to your weight anymore. Instead, you can focus on living your life to the fullest and thrive. At the same time, the changes to your body become automated too. You will discover a way of living that allows your body to function correctly, meaning you won't always have to look at food labels or count calories. It's time for me to outline the chapters that will come together to create your roadmap to success. Weight loss is achieved easily when you learn to motivate the Elephant and become a good Rider.

Motivate The Elephant

The goal is to motivate the Elephant and use its sheer power to drive you in the direction you wish to go in. This isn't achieved by burying your head in the sand and dismissing your emotions. Instead, it would be best if you learned from them. Negative emotions are normal. We all experience sadness, anger, emptiness, fear, guilt, failure and resentment. There are many other negative emotions we all experience throughout our lives too. We should never be ashamed to feel these emotions. We should never be afraid to talk about them either. Life works best when you understand them. When you notice how you feel and act because of them. Doing this will teach you how to deal with certain situations and discover patterns in your life and emotional decision-making. If you don't take notice of your emotions, you will let them control you, often making achieving your goal more difficult.

There are three chapters to motivate the Elephant. The first is Grow Yourself. Within this chapter, I introduce you to the three pillars of growing yourself - Grow Your Mindset, Improve Your Eating Habits, and Be More Active. These three pillars allow you to cultivate a sense of identity in your way of eating and lifestyle, helping you decide what's best for you. The first pillar encourages you to develop a growth mindset, helping you achieve your weight loss goal more confidently. All of this motivates the Elephant as it will feel as though it's improving and can see no limitations to the foods it can consume. It feels as though its feelings are being factored in.

THE ELEPHANT AND THE RIDER

The first chapter provides the Elephant with the knowledge it needs to be motivated to begin initially heading in the right direction, yet knowing something isn't enough to cause change. Find The Feeling is the second chapter, split into two parts, and will be the most motivating to the Elephant. A weight loss goal isn't achieved by focusing on the number it says on the scales. It is achieved by having a strong emotional connection to your weight loss journey that will be with it every step of the way. It's also the chapter where you will set clear motivational goals to fuel your journey further. You will also set behavioural goals, so the Elephant knows precisely how to act and is happy with the clear actions set in this chapter. The second part of Find The Feeling encourages you to find something you love. When you do this, you will be happy with new ways of being more active and living a healthier lifestyle.

We often try to make many changes at once, but the Elephant doesn't like this. Shrink The Change helps you break down the required changes so it doesn't spook the Elephant. Instead, this chapter encourages you to focus on making your changes so small that the Elephant doesn't even notice them. This motivates the Elephant as it feels change is possible. Every small change you gradually make motivates the Elephant more and more. Before you know it, the Elephant is running to your weight loss goal, taking the Rider with them.

Learn To Be A Good Rider

A motivated elephant is the driving force behind your weight loss journey. Once it gets going, it will be travelling at speed. The Elephant can easily be distracted, just like a dog to a squirrel, biscuit, or ball. The last thing you want is to be sat on top of an elephant that's chasing its tail. It would be best if you made the road as Roman as possible. To do this, you must learn how to become a good rider to keep the Elephant's powerful motivation charging straight towards your weight loss destination. Just like motivating the Elephant, three chapters will help you do this.

The first chapter in becoming a good rider is to find your bright spots. We often focus on the things we aren't doing well, which begins any journey of self-improvement with negative thoughts. To become a good rider, you must look at what you're already doing well in your life. These are known as bright spots. In this chapter, you will investigate what you're already doing well and clone these actions to allow weight loss to be achieved easily. When you do this, you begin with positive thoughts and feelings, and the Elephant and the Rider will follow the road of least resistance.

Earlier, I mentioned shrinking the change where you make small changes to allow the Elephant to feel change is possible. If change was left to the Elephant, it would make one hundred changes at once or none at all. The changes it would decide to make wouldn't be beneficial. We often sweat the small stuff and spend all our time focusing on the things that don't matter too much. The

THE ELEPHANT AND THE RIDER

Elephant gets distracted by fads, trends, and friends, so you need to filter the many possible changes you could make to become a good Rider. This is known as scripting your critical moves. The second chapter on becoming a good Rider encourages you to make the most significant change first and to always focus on making just one change at a time.

By the third chapter, you will have gained control of the Elephant. Not in a forceful way, but one that the Elephant is happy with. The final thing to do to learn how to become a good Rider is to ensure the Elephant is pointing to the destination. Once you know where you are currently, where you want to go, and why you wish to get to the destination, there's only one thing left: How do you get there? The last thing you want to do is charge off in the wrong direction. The third chapter is split in two.

The first part will help you plan your journey in advance. Instead of reacting to a situation and allowing the Elephant to make an emotional decision, you plan accordingly. This is done by anticipating potential barriers and thinking about how to overcome them. Planning ahead takes all the stress, worries, and bad decisions out of your journey. Change is easier when you know what you're doing and where you're going. The Rider is much happier when they can see a clear road that makes sense to follow.

The second part of Point To The Destination is Planning Your Meals. Here, you will use the knowledge gained from Improve Your Eating Habits to plan your meals in a way you're happy. You will be shown how to portion out each food group to prevent over-eating and encouraged to consider which part of your day requires further improvement. You're almost ready to go once you've Pointed To The Destination.

The Rider is sitting on top of the Elephant, and the lights are on amber. There's one thing left before the lights turn green: Shape The Road. This chapter stands alone and makes the road you're about to follow clearer and easier. People often set off on their weight loss journey knowing there will be resistance from their loved ones, current habits, and the general environment. Shape The Road sets the Elephant and the Rider up for success, clearing any potential resistance from your environment. In this chapter, you will tweak your environment to create one on your side, strengthen your support structure, and learn how to build new habits. The final chapter in this book is Ride Into The Sunset. Everything you've learnt in this book and created action plans for will be used to create your weight loss roadmap. Once you've checked and confirmed your actions, the lights turn green, and the Elephant and the Rider are ready to Ride Into The Sunset.

Learn From The Past

Now that you understand what the Elephant and the Rider are and how they will help you throughout the remaining chapters, I wish to close this chapter by learning from the past. Many people search for new ways of losing weight, yet they don't stop to think for a second about their past. All humans are capable of looking introspectively at their own experiences, allowing us to interpret how we feel, think, and act. When we do this, we can use the knowledge gained from these previous experiences to help ourselves improve in the future. This is why you need to reflect on the past. Learning comes not only from doing but from thinking about what we do. The more you can learn from your previous actions, the easier it will be to succeed in the future.

The Elephant hates failure, but that doesn't mean you should avoid it. We all often fail at things, as failure is a part of life. This is why you need to create the expectation of failure, not failure of your weight loss journey, but potential failure on the route. The Rider knows this, which is why it's important to learn how to become a good Rider. When you do this, you can tame the Elephant's emotions so that when it experiences failure, it's no longer fazed. Your previous failures let you know what you could do differently next time. When you reflect on the past, you will soon realise where the Elephant's fear of failure has taken you off course. You will see the times the Rider could've steered the Elephant back on track. This section is a learning curve which will allow the Elephant and the Rider to improve the quality of their weight-loss journey.

Reflection allows you to take control of your future. It will enable you to gain helpful information that's specific to you. This allows you to personalise your future actions, which creates sustainable change. You will build a stronger connection between yourself and your body. The more you can understand your own actions, who you are as a person, and how your body works, the easier controlling your weight will be. It may seem strange, but reflecting is a way of getting to know yourself. You will see how your emotions are, what you're good at, what you aren't so good at, and you will also see how you respond to certain situations.

The better connected you are to yourself, the clearer your actions become. In doing this, you are less likely to fail in the future. You learn where you went wrong and what you could do to prevent that situation from happening again. This is why you are less likely to fail in the future if you reflect regularly. As you are less likely to fail, you are more likely to succeed. You are constantly evolving and improving if you reflect regularly. There are some people stuck in a rut for all of their lives. These people aren't reflecting on how they can improve. Preventing them from seeing what needs to change to allow them to evolve into successful people.

You can now see that reflection is crucial in helping you move forward, achieve your weight loss goal, and keep the weight off. You must ensure you keep your reflection on point. If you have a short attention span or an overthinking mind, you may veer away from reflecting on your previous weight loss attempts and struggles. One reflection question can lead to many other questions, like one YouTube video can send you down a rabbit hole. Before you know it, you are thinking about why you wore that crazy outfit to your friend's birthday twenty years ago. It's great that a question leads to another question as it shows that your reflecting skills are on point, but write down the next question and continue focussing on the current one before you move on. Some diversions can lead to fantastic reflection sessions. Yet, some can just as easily go on to completely different topics, providing you with no value at all. Maintain focus by bringing it back to the point.

When reflecting, you can learn and grow or dwell and say no. It doesn't matter what has happened in your past, so don't beat yourself up if you think of a negative thought or situation. Instead, the idea is to learn from it and say, "This happened, and it didn't work, but what I will do next time is…". If you are starting to think negatively about your past, I advise you to take some time to process what you've reflected so far. In doing so, you allow time to help you make sense of the situation and see how it will help you in the future. If you're ready, then answer the first question.

What has brought you to this very point?

There are many reasons why people search for something to help them. You don't know where to start. You may feel overwhelmed by the vast amount of information out there. Some are frustrated with trying to achieve their goals and being unable to reach them. Others are stuck in the world of yoyo dieting, and their weight has fluctuated for years. Then, there are those who have been searching for long-term, sustainable lifestyle changes. There are so many reasons why you could be reading this page right now. What has brought you to this very point today?

- Have you had a health scare?
- Are you sick and tired of feeling sick and tired?
- Has something big happened?
- Have you just thought enough is enough?
- Have you hit a milestone birthday and shit yourself?

Each individual moves through three stages before they take action. Pre-contemplation is the stage where people have no interest in taking action as they're unaware their behaviour is problematic. In this stage, people underestimate the pros of making a change and cement beliefs about the cons. The Elephant is scared of failing, and the Rider is nowhere to be seen. The second stage a person goes through is Contemplation, where people begin to talk about potentially losing weight. They begin to recognise their behaviour is problematic and start to think about the pros and cons of taking action, ending up with mixed feelings. The Elephant still fears change, but the Rider has thrown on the saddle. The third stage is Preparation, where people begin to make small steps towards making a change. Purchasing this book is part of the preparation stage. They plan to take action within the next thirty days. The Elephant is open to change, and the Rider jumps on board.

Everything within this book is about getting the Elephant and The Rider prepared to take the action needed to achieve your weight loss goal. To do this, you take the actions required at the end of each chapter. This stage is where people modify their behaviour, intending to

THE ELEPHANT AND THE RIDER

keep progressing. I'm sure you've got to this stage many times before. In the past, the Rider has tried controlling the Elephant too hard and forced it to take actions it didn't want to. This has led to a relapse and is the cause of weight gain. As you know by now, the key to sustainable change is to factor in both the Elephant and the Rider. Change only sticks when both of them are happy with the changes you are making. If you're lucky enough to keep control of the Elephant long enough, you might end up at the maintenance stage. This is where you've achieved your weight loss goal and wish to keep the weight off. The Elephant and The Rider have worked together and are still happy. People in this stage work to prevent relapses and continue living a healthy life.

The final stage is termination. If you reach this stage, you will have achieved your weight loss goal, kept the weight off for at least six months, and have no desire to return to old habits and behaviours. As they are sure they won't relapse, they no longer have to keep track of their food intake, worry about their weight, or continue making changes. Instead, their life runs on autopilot, and all the healthy actions required are completed subconsciously. People rarely make it to the termination stage and those who think they do tend to skip the maintenance stage and terminate prematurely. It's essential to be in the maintenance stage for at least six months before intentionally terminating.

Now I've explained the six stages of change, I want to ask the following questions.

1. When did you move from pre-contemplation to contemplation, and why?
2. When did you move from contemplation to preparation, and why?
3. Have you ever moved from preparation to action without factoring in the emotions of the Elephant?

When you think about what has brought you to this very sentence, you will see a chain of events leading to this point. Reflecting allows you to see this and gain a greater insight into your actions and behaviours so far. After reflecting on these questions, I want you to think about what you can learn from the reasons you've wanted to change. Why you have moved from pre-contemplation to preparation, and whether you're ready to move to the action stage. As the goal is for the Elephant and the Rider to work together, it's crucial to think about your emotions.

What hasn't worked in the past?

Reflecting on your emotions begins with asking yourself, "What hasn't worked in the past?" I need you to think long and hard about every single way you've attempted to lose weight. It could have been a specific diet, a workout plan, a gym membership, something a friend told you to do, or even another book you've read. Once you've written down all the previous ways, you need to consider why it didn't work for you. It's crazy how we all do things, decide it's not for us, and stop doing it. I'm sure you've been to an exercise class once and once only. Back in the day, I used to run bootcamps and would see people come once, never to be seen again. I always wondered why that was, but did they? Maybe it was too hard for them or somehow too easy. They might have felt intimidated or self-conscious exercising with sixty other people. Perhaps it was because they hated me and thought I was a rubbish instructor. Regardless, there was a reason why they were never to be seen again.

I need you to think of why you stopped following a diet, ended your gym membership, or gave up trying to lose weight. It's important to look at your previous experiences as evidence rather than failures. Each time you've tried something, you have collected data that can be used to plan your future. As you're about to create a way of losing weight that will work for you, collecting as much data as possible would be valuable. It's time to look at all the things you've tried in the past.

- What diets have you tried?
- Which types of exercise have you tried?
- Why do you think they haven't worked for you?
- How did you feel whilst you were following them?

It's easy to slip back into doing something you've tried in the past as it's something you're familiar with. The Elephant doesn't like change. It knows these methods don't work, yet it resorts back to them as some form of safety blanket. This is where the logical Rider needs to pull them out of the trap of the quick fix, big change, or trendy plan they've both tried in the past. The easiest way of

THE ELEPHANT AND THE RIDER

getting out of this trap is to ask yourself this question for each weight loss method you've tried in the past: How did that work for me?

- Did a restrictive diet work for you long-term?
- Did that crazy workout plan turn you into a Greek god?

Or

- Did the restrictive diet make you feel sad, starving, and want to binge eat?
- Did the crazy workout plan get dismissed after the first week because it was too hard and time-consuming?

When you ask yourself how previous weight loss attempts have worked for you, it can be tempting to think of the short-term results some gave you. There's no point in losing weight to gaining it back, so you need to think about how it worked for you in the long term. The next time you try to lose weight will be the last. You must remove any temptation to chase short-term results by repeating previous weight loss methods. You know the type of person you are. Did your previous methods factor in your personality? You know how much time you have to cook and exercise. Did you have enough time, or were you short on time? You know what intensity you're willing to work at. Was it too intense for you? You know the lifestyle you live. Were they sustainable methods for you? Most importantly, you know how you feel while following a specific exercise plan or diet. Were you happy or unhappy? Interested or bored? Able to socialise or be isolated instead?

The final part of reflection is to think about what your previous experiences are telling you. There's no point in reflecting on things and not processing them. Having a list of previous ways of losing weight is pointless if you haven't gained valuable information from reflecting on them. What does all of this information tell you? This book encourages you to decide what to do based on the results you get. Have your previous choices given you the results you want? If they helped you lose weight, did they allow you to keep it off? If the answer to these questions is no, maybe it's time to chuck them in room 101. The answers to most questions often lie in our ability to reflect on what has failed us and why. Reflection prevents us from making the same mistakes again. You also realise what you've been lacking, such as a plan that puts you in the driving seat or factors in both the Elephant and the Rider.

Your To-Do List

1. Reflect on the past and consider what you could learn from it that would help you in the future.
2. Ask yourself if you're a good rider. Consider whether you're currently making logical decisions and have control of the Elephant.
3. Ask yourself if you're motivating the Elephant. Think about whether you motivate the Elephant or

THE ELEPHANT AND THE RIDER

are strict and punish it. Do you factor in your emotions when trying to lose weight?

4

TRACK YOUR FOOD INTAKE

What gets measured gets managed. If your finances need reviewing, you first download your bank statements and look at ways you can save. How much are you earning? How much are you spending? What are you spending too much money on? You begin to track your spending habits to ensure you have enough money in the bank to cover your bills. You put aside some money each month to take the family on holiday in twelve months—budgeting for an amazing experience and lifelong memories further down the line.

You can't achieve this if you don't track your finances, and you can't guarantee weight loss if you don't track your food intake. The word I've just used there is guarantee. If you lose weight by tracking your food intake, you guarantee that weight loss will occur, so why risk it by not tracking? If you're going to put the effort into losing weight, then you want results, don't you?

Tracking your food intake consists of three parts: Calories, Macronutrients, and Food choices. The first I need to discuss is calories. Calories are the energy you consume through food and burn off through bodily functions and movement. You don't need to know the ins and outs of calories; you just need to think of them as money. You get a certain amount to spend each day, and it's up to you what you decide to use them on. Some people like to have three big meals and no snacks. Others prefer to have two regular meals and two snacks. Some consume fewer calories than they need throughout the week, so they can spend a few more over the weekend. You can spend them however you wish. All you need to be aware of is the outline below.

- When you take in more calories than your body burns - You **gain** weight.
- When you take in the same calories as your body burns - You **maintain** weight.
- When you take in fewer calories than your body burns - You **lose** weight.

Your weight is all about energy balance, measured by your calories. To lose weight, you must consume fewer calories than your body burns. It's that simple. Tracking your food intake allows you to see if this is the case. Calories in vs calories out is the fundamental concept of body weight regulation and is as close to scientific fact as possible. You

TRACK YOUR FOOD INTAKE

can't argue with it. Every time you've lost weight in the past, it is because whatever method you've used has put you in a calorie deficit.

It doesn't matter if it was through fasting, cutting out a food group, or counting your points; you lost weight because you were consuming fewer calories than your body needed. For now, ignore everything around you and understand the most crucial action you need to take to guarantee weight loss: tracking your calories to ensure you're in a calorie deficit. You don't need to do it forever; over time, you will learn how many calories are in the foods you're consuming and how much food that is.

Chapter 1 outlined the ten main reasons you think weight loss is hard. You also know the purpose of this book is to show you that weight loss isn't as hard as you think. Tracking your calorie intake eliminates seven of the reasons you believe weight loss is hard. Consume fewer calories than your body needs, and you will lose weight. This is the clear direction you need. All diets work the same by putting you in a calorie deficit. No conflicting messages are here, so you don't need to resort to extremes. By tracking your calories, you will be in complete control without the restrictions you're used to. You decide what you spend your calories on, giving you freedom and flexibility on your weight loss journey. You will also see that you don't need to drop your calories or food intake too low to lose weight.

You can feel in control without the restriction. This means you won't have to be hard on yourself because even if you have a glass of wine or a dessert, you will see

TRACK YOUR FOOD INTAKE

the numbers and be able to balance the books. You can enjoy it rather than feel guilty about it. You remain in a happy place and on track because you can clearly see if you will be in a calorie deficit. If you're not, no worries; you consume slightly fewer calories over the forthcoming days to balance the books, and you will still lose weight. There's no need to be hard on yourself, preventing dieting from messing with the body and mind. You will be happy with the simplicity and freedom you have been provided with. You won't always feel starving, low on energy, or like a failure.

Tracking your calories is the most straightforward plan you need to lose weight. Remember, simplicity is the ultimate sophistication. Obviously, we will bolster this plan throughout the book, but your plan starts here. The plan is to track your calorie intake to ensure you guarantee weight loss. By following this simple plan, you will no longer feel exhausted trying to lose weight. You will clearly know whether you will lose weight or not by tracking your calorie intake. The plan is simple, and the message is clear: track your calorie intake, and you will lose weight. Weight loss isn't as hard as you think.

Now that you understand the importance of tracking your calories, you must know how many calories you should consume. The recommended daily amount of calories to maintain weight is 2,000 calories for women and 2,500 calories for men. The main reason men's recommended calorie intake is 500 greater is that most men have greater muscle mass than women, and muscle requires more calories to maintain than body fat. If you're female and want to eat more, get lifting some weights and build some muscle mass. If you are male and sitting at a desk all day, your recommended daily calorie intake would likely be lower than 2500 as you won't have much muscle mass compared to a male on a building site.

If you wish to lose weight, you need to be in a calorie deficit, meaning you consume less calories than your body needs. The recommended amount of calories to reduce is 500 calories daily, which would take your daily calorie intake to 1500 calories for a woman and 2000 for a man. One pound of body fat equals 3500 calories, meaning you must consume 3500 calories less than you need to lose it. It also means to gain one pound of body fat you must consume 3500 calories more than your body needs to maintain weight. 500 calories multiplied by seven days equals 3500. This is the most sustainable way of losing body fat, as one pound per week is a realistic amount. That being said, it doesn't mean you can't lose more, especially at the beginning of your weight loss journey, and this is all because of your basal metabolic rate, which I discussed earlier in chapter three. To recap, this is the number of calories you burn as your body performs functions to keep you alive. It's how many calories you burn if you stay in bed all day, and the greater your weight is, the higher your BMR is. The simplest way to work out your basal metabolic rate is below.

Basal Metabolic Rate = Weight in KG x 24

TRACK YOUR FOOD INTAKE

- If you weigh 120kg, multiply it by 24 for a BMR of 2880 calories.
- If you weigh 100kg, multiply it by 24 for a BMR of 2400 calories.
- If you weigh 80kg, multiply it by 24 for a BMR of 1920 calories.
- If you weigh 60kg, multiply it by 24 for a BMR of 1440 calories.

As you can see, the more you weigh, the more calories you need to function. This is why people who weigh more tend to lose more at the beginning of their weight loss journey, as their deficit will be greater if they follow the recommendations of consuming 1500 calories per day to lose weight. It's also why people's weight loss feels as though it's plateauing as their weight drops; they don't adjust their daily calorie requirements in line with how much they weigh.

- If you consume 1500 calories daily and weigh 120kg, you will lose 4 pounds of body fat in one week.
- If you consume 1500 calories daily and weigh 100kg, you will lose 2.75 pounds of body fat in one week.
- If you consume 1500 calories daily and weigh 80kg, you will lose 1.6 pounds of body fat in one week

TRACK YOUR FOOD INTAKE

- If you consume 1500 calories daily and weigh 60kg, you will lose 0.5 pounds of body fat in one week.

This means you only need to drop your calorie intake to 1500 calories if you weigh 80kg or less. If you currently weigh over 80kg, you don't have to drop your daily calorie intake to 1500 calories if you don't want to. You can still lose weight, but it will be slower. The leap from 2880 calories daily to 1500 calories can feel too big. If you drop your calories somewhere in the middle, you will still lose two pounds of body fat in one week. Conversely, a person who is 60kg and wishes to drop weight will find it challenging as they would have to consume 1228 calories per day to lose one pound of body fat. This can be a tricky feat as it means consuming a low amount of calories each day. It's always best in these situations to lower your expectations and aim to lose 0.5 pounds of body fat in one week by consuming 1500 calories each day. Just understand that when you start your weight loss journey, you will lose more than you will further down the line; it's completely normal.

Tracking your food intake also shows you the macronutrients in them. Macronutrients are carbohydrates, fats, and proteins. They are the nutrients we need in large quantities that provide energy in the form of calories. I won't go into the roles of each macronutrient just yet, as this chapter is about tracking your food intake. They are all needed for your body to function correctly, and remember, when your body functions correctly, weight loss and weight control are more effortless. Before I go into the guidelines for macronutrients, I need you to understand that the most important part of tracking your food intake right now is tracking your calorie intake. This is a book, so I must explain everything to you right now. Don't worry too much about everything I'm about to explain, as it can seem like a lot.

One gram of carbohydrates and one gram of protein contains four calories each. One gram of fat contains nine calories. This is why fat seems to have a bad reputation, as it's higher in calories than carbohydrates and protein, but you don't need as much of it. Generally, you would aim to consume 1.5g of protein per kilogram of body weight. This is because you want to maintain any muscle mass that you currently have. Muscles are a good weight as they require a lot of calories to maintain and make you look toned. If you weigh 80kg, 120g of protein is recommended daily, which means 480 calories per day from protein. The rest, in all honesty, is your call. Some people prefer consuming more fats, while others prefer more carbohydrates. The guideline for fat consumption has been 0.5-1g per kg of body weight which would equate to 360 to 720 calories. The rationale for this is that some weight loss studies indicate that people who had more success in losing and maintaining weight consumed less than one gram of fat per kg of body weight per day. If you followed these guidelines, it would leave 300-660 calories daily from carbohydrates.

As well as macronutrients, tracking your food intake lets you know where most of your food intake comes from

TRACK YOUR FOOD INTAKE

regarding breakfast, lunch, dinner, and snacks. This allows you to see which parts of your food intake are going well for you and which require altering to help you lose weight. You're collecting valuable data to help you on your weight loss journey. It may sound like a pain in the backside, but I will provide you with a simple way to get all of this data with the click of a button.

You now know that weight loss is as simple as calories in versus calories out; you must consume fewer calories than your body needs. To ensure you are doing this, you must track your food intake to see how many calories and nutrients are in your food and drinks. You will be able to see patterns that may be helping or hindering your weight loss progress, allowing you to be more aware of your eating habits. Often, we're unaware of how many calories are in the foods we eat, especially the packaged items. By being able to see the amount of calories you're consuming, the types of food you're eating, and the patterns in your eating habits, you can then make the changes needed. I cannot stress how important this is when you're trying to lose weight. Do you now see tracking your food intake is crucial to guarantee weight loss? Are you happy to begin tracking your food intake?

If that's not swaying you, think of your emotions. There's nothing more frustrating than not knowing where you've been going wrong, is there? Think of all the times you've tried to lose weight in the past and been left wondering why you were unsuccessful and blaming yourself instead. That's the last thing we want. Tracking your food intake gets rid of that confusion. It allows you to

TRACK YOUR FOOD INTAKE

see the picture in a thousand calories. You no longer blame yourself because instead of wondering why, you can see the story. You can control the ending by looking at what's going on, preventing the blame game from kicking in. Instead of negative emotions taking over your mind, you feel empowered and in control. Nothing is going to stop you this time. You know where you're going wrong. You know what needs to change. There's no "I'm destined to be this way for the rest of my life" renditions. Instead, you know you've got this.

Trying to lose weight without tracking your food intake is a gamble. The odds are stacked against you. Have you ever put a bet on the Grand National? This annual event involves forty horses participating in a long race over thirty challenging fences. Fence by fence, horses fall, and only a handful make it over the finish line. Throughout your weight loss journey, you must ensure you don't fall at any fences and make it over the finish line. Tracking your food intake allows you to measure your performance to anticipate the end result. What gets measured gets managed. If you don't track, you don't know whether you will lose weight, gain some or stay the same. You won't know whether you will make it over the finish line.

Some people would argue that tracking your calories doesn't work. It does work; however, there are a few things you need to understand. For some silly reason, food labels are allowed to be incorrect. According to FDA guidelines, they can be up to 20% inaccurate. There's not much we, as the public, can do about this absurdity. Earlier, I spoke about your Basal Metabolic Rate (BMR). The amount of

TRACK YOUR FOOD INTAKE

recommended calories to consume tends to be your BMR multiplied by 1.2. As you can see, the calculation adds 20% to your BMR to account for calories burnt off through food digestion, activity and exercise. The easiest thing we can do if food labels are up to 20% inaccurate is not to add the recommended 20% calorie intake to our BMR. This way, the 20% inaccuracy through food labels has been cancelled out by us not adding 20% to our BMR. This is why, earlier on, I only told you to work out your BMR, and I didn't mention the extra 20%. This is the best thing we can do to ensure that tracking your food intake guarantees weight loss success. Although it isn't 100% accurate, we have taken action to ensure it is as close as possible.

Another reason why people may argue that tracking your calories doesn't work is because they aren't tracking correctly. For this to work, you must track and log everything that passes your lips. This includes a bite off your kid's plate, the chocolate passed around the office, and the liquids you consume. It doesn't matter whether it's a 'good' or 'bad' food or fluid; you must track it all. There's no point in only logging the good stuff. What's the point in that? If you log everything you consume, you will lose weight and stay on track to achieving your weight loss goal. Continuing from this, the final thing to say is you need to be consistent for this to work. Just like only tracking the good stuff, there's no point in only logging Monday to Friday. You need to track everything you consume every single day. It may be a pain to begin with, but it will be easier once you get into the swing of things. Remember why you're doing this and the importance of tracking your food intake.

How do I track my food intake?

If you're left scratching your head and believing you need to crunch numbers on a calculator and put them on a spreadsheet, don't worry. There's an app for everything these days, and in the modern world, we are glued to our smartphones. This is why the easiest way to track your food intake is with a free app called MyFitnessPal. This app will record your calories, macronutrients and food choices with the click of a button. It records every piece of data related to your food intake, which is one powerful thing. There is every food you can think of within it, with 14 million in its database. Once you get into the habit of clicking on the app each time you eat or drink something, it will be effortless and automated. It certainly beats having to calorie count by reading the labels and logging them in a journal like the good old days.

I'm going to explain everything you need to do. It would help if you had your phone out and followed the steps as we go through the next few paragraphs. The first thing you need to do is download MyFitnessPal from the App Store on your phone. When you first open the app, it will ask you to sign up using your email address or social media log-in. You only need the free app, so don't pay for the paid version. The free version has everything you need, so you might as well save the pennies. It will then ask you to create a username. Once you're signed up, it will ask you

TRACK YOUR FOOD INTAKE

to enter your starting weight. Jump on the scales to get your starting weight. Don't worry about what it says; what matters is what it says in the future.

Once you've logged your starting weight, you must log your goal weight; This is the weight that you would ultimately like to be. You are then asked to enter your weekly goal; This is how much weight you wish to lose each week. You will see that it doesn't exceed two pounds per week. This is because two pounds per week is the maximum body fat you can hit consistently. There may be times when you lose more, especially at the beginning of your weight loss journey. There will be times on your journey where half a pound lost in one week is fantastic. But your weekly target can be no more than two pounds lost weekly. Finally, you are asked for your activity levels. If you have an office job, select not very active. If you have an active job, select not active or active. I'd avoid selecting very active for now, even if you are. This is because MyFitnessPal will increase your daily calorie intake, which may prevent you from losing weight. If you are very active, select this once you achieve your weight loss goal and want to maintain your weight.

Once you've set up MyFitnessPal, you need to know how to use it. Searching for food may feel like a pain initially, but this is the most important new habit you can acquire. It will also get easier and quicker to log your food intake the more you do it. At the bottom of the page, there is a plus symbol. Click on this and select food. It will then ask if you wish to add it for breakfast, lunch, dinner, or a snack. Click on the required meal to add your food. Once

TRACK YOUR FOOD INTAKE

you've selected the meal you want to log, you must search for the food or foods you eat. At the top of the page, there is a search box. Enter the foods you wish to log.

Once you've logged something once, it will be on there for good, so if you eat the same thing regularly, it will be waiting for you in your history the next time you consume it. Once you've found your food, click on the tick symbol at the top of the page to save it. After you've logged your food, it will take you to your food diary, where you can see your calories and food intake for that particular day.

There are many features within MyFitnessPal that you need to know about. The first is how to log your weight. It would be best to only step on the scales once per week as this allows you to focus on the actions needed rather than the end result. If you weigh yourself multiple times per week, you're just adding stress to your life. Weigh yourself first thing in the morning after going to the toilet. This is the most reliable time to weigh, as your weight naturally fluctuates throughout the day due to fluid and food intake. All you need to do to log your weight is press the plus symbol and select weight to log your new weight. As I mentioned earlier, the lighter you are, the fewer calories your body needs, which is why it's important to log your weight on MyFitnessPal, as it will adjust your daily calorie target accordingly.

The next thing to cover is your weekly calorie intake. This is a fantastic feature as it looks at the bigger picture. It shows your weekly calorie goal, which is your daily calorie goal multiplied by seven. This allows you to see whether you're on track for the week. We are often stuck

TRACK YOUR FOOD INTAKE

sweating the small stuff, such as going over your daily calorie intake by two hundred calories on a Monday. If this happens, you can adjust the remaining days to stay under your weekly calorie goal. The same goes for the weekends. If you've got a busy weekend coming up, you can bank some calories each weekday so you have more to use over the weekend. Taking off two hundred calories Monday to Friday will provide you with an additional thousand calories over the weekend. This allows you to have a few beers or go out for dinner and still lose weight. You will lose weight if you don't go over your weekly calorie goal. It doesn't matter if you have the same amount each day or have less throughout the weekdays to have more over the weekend. It's your life, your weight loss journey, so spend them as you choose. At the bottom of the app is a tab labelled More. Click here and select 'Nutrition' from the menu at the top of the page. Select calories, then click on day view to change it to weekly view. Here, you will see your weekly calories total.

    The final feature allows you to see the types of foods you're consuming. This is something I will cover later in greater detail. As mentioned earlier, macronutrients are protein, fats, and carbohydrates, and we should be consuming specific quantities of each to allow our bodies to function efficiently. The main focus of tracking your food intake is ensuring you lose weight by tracking your calories. Still, macronutrients come in at a close second. Checking out your weekly macronutrient consumption is the same process as finding your weekly calories. Click the 'More' tab in the bottom corner, click 'Nutrition', and select 'Macros' at the top. Here, you can see how much of your diet consists of carbs, fats and proteins.

Within this section, you can also alter your goal for each type of macronutrient, which is helpful. Earlier, I stated that you should aim for 1.5g of protein per kilogram of body weight. If you weigh 80kg, then that would be 120g. Where it says a percentage 'Goal' next to protein, click on it to change the percentage to one that shows 120g. You can also do this for fats to show 0.5g of fat per kg of body weight, so if you weigh 80kg, then slide the fat percentage to one that shows 40g. Finally, place whatever percentage you have left for carbohydrates so the total percentage equals 100%.

What about diets?

I bet in your mind you've had a voice that keeps chirping away at you. One that's reminding you of the word I'm trying not to mention. Am I Right? Is the voice saying, "He hasn't mentioned the word diet"? The inner voice is trying to alarm you to something, so I'd best challenge it and explain why I'm not mentioning the word diet. To commit to something, you need to understand it, something most people can't do with diets. It doesn't matter how each diet is branded or packaged. It doesn't matter what structure it has, whether fasting, taking out food groups, or eating a specific food. They all work by doing the same thing: putting you in a calorie deficit and encouraging you to consume less energy than your body needs. I wish for you to do what you wish to do. To eat the foods you wish to eat. To lose weight in a way that suits you and your needs. I want you to be in control, not a diet. I want you to have choice, not restriction. I want you to feel like you're not actually on a diet because you're not; you're following a way of eating that's going to allow you to control your weight for the rest of your life.

I haven't mentioned the word diet so far because you go on and off a diet, meaning there's a beginning and an end. A diet works at the beginning, and you can lose weight, but you can't sustain it, so it ends, and the weight creeps back up. It's a method of misery and sacrifice for short-term gain. Losing weight without following a diet and instead tracking your food intake is the long-term solution. If you went on a diet for three months, you still have many years to live, meaning you will be stuck in the diet trap and repeatedly be on or off a diet. Instead, find a way of eating that will allow you to lose weight and then control your weight once you get there.

I spoke about our body's hunger and fullness hormones, Leptin and Ghrelin, in the Understanding Body Weight chapter. We don't speak about or understand the various hormones in the body. Occasionally, someone may speak about insulin because they have diabetes or mention a thyroid issue. Still, many hormones play essential roles in various bodily functions. Your body functions at its best when you provide everything it needs. This involves fats, carbs, proteins, vitamins and minerals, water, and sleep, among other things. Diets forget about them, which has a negative impact on your physical and mental well-being.

Leptin and Ghrelin decide whether you will lose or gain weight due to playing a role in your weight set point. Diets don't address your weight set point and instead act like a bull in a china shop. They want you to rush around and lose as much weight as possible in the shortest time. Altering your way of eating and gradually decreasing your body weight allows you to lose weight and lower your weight set point over time, allowing you to lose weight and keep it off.

You now understand why I'm not pushing a specific diet. Your body functions at its best when you aren't on one. The final reason why I'm encouraging you to eat, not diet, is because diets are too restrictive. They have fixed rules, such as only eating certain food groups or at certain times of the day. Food is fuel so you can thrive and survive, but it's also there to be enjoyed too. A sustainable approach allows celebrations, enjoyment, and a treat or two. Life is flexible, and eating should be fluid. A flexible approach to your eating habits is essential for long-term results.

If you wish to follow a specific diet, that's fine; you can do that. This book is about helping you make your own decisions and decide what is best for you. Just understand that it's not an essential part of the weight loss process, so if you don't want to go on a diet, you don't have to. All you need to do is track your food intake and ensure you're in a calorie deficit.

TRACK YOUR FOOD INTAKE

Don't Drop Your Calorie Intake Too Low

The dieting world means you're used to speedy weight loss. The unrealistic and unsustainable results of unhealthy weight loss methods. When losing weight, dropping your calorie intake to low numbers can be tempting. The belief that fewer calories means quicker results leads people to search for short-term gratification, only to be stung further down the line. Low numbers are down to three, four, or five hundred calories daily to try and lose weight faster. You've purchased this book to lose weight, but I'm sure you wanted to be healthy too? I'm also sure you wish to keep the weight off that you're going to lose.

The most crucial reason why you should never drop your calorie intake too low is because of your vital organs. They're called vital organs, as they are those that a person needs to survive. A problem with any of these organs can quickly become life-threatening. They are your heart, brain, lungs, liver and kidneys, and they need plenty of energy in the form of calories to function. Your heart's function is to keep blood flowing through the body. Blood also carries substances that cells need and takes away waste. Your brain functions as the body's control centre. It controls thoughts, memories, emotions, touch, motor skills, vision, breathing, temperature, hunger, and every process that regulates your body. Your lung's primary function is breathing, exchanging oxygen and carbon dioxide with the blood. Your kidneys filter blood and form urine, which is then excreted from the body. Your liver

TRACK YOUR FOOD INTAKE

filters blood, secretes bile needed for digestion, and produces proteins necessary for blood clotting.

You must provide your body with a certain amount of calories to complete these vital bodily functions. Earlier, I spoke about your Basal Metabolic Rate (BMR), which is how many calories your body needs to function daily. All those calories needed for your body to function each day are vital, and you must be consuming the required amount to ensure you look after your body. If you don't consume sufficient calories because you're tempted to lose weight quicker, please understand that you can cause irreversible damage. Your brain needs four hundred calories per day. Your heart and lungs combined need four hundred calories. Your liver and kidneys, together, require four hundred calories per day, too. This is why you should never drop your calorie intake any lower than twelve hundred calories. Don't be tempted to follow diets that promote daily calorie consumption any lower than twelve hundred. Your vital organs need them daily to work at their best and keep you alive and well.

The dangerous thing about dropping your calorie intake too low is that your vital organs adapt. Let's say you're not consuming the twelve hundred calories daily that your vital organs need. Instead, you only consume six hundred per day for a prolonged time. What happens then is your vital organs adapt. They assume they will no longer receive the total energy they need. Instead, they will only get fifty per cent, six hundred calories. Based on this, they need to adapt and run at a lower capacity. This means your heart, lungs, brain, liver and kidneys no longer work as well as they used to. As I mentioned earlier, you're causing irreversible damage to these vital organs. The last thing you want is heart disease. The last thing you want is for your liver and kidneys to be unable to flush out toxins from the body. The last thing you want is difficulty breathing or a brain that doesn't remember, control movement, or make decisions as well as it should. I apologise if this sounds intimidating; it's dangerous if you drop your calorie intake too low, and I needed to explain to you why. The last thing you want is health complications.

Like most diets, dropping your calorie intake too low isn't sustainable; you won't be able to stick to it. You will hate it as you will always be starving, so you shouldn't drop your calories to unsustainable levels. When you're starving all the time, your hunger hormone Ghrelin starts kicking in. Because you've been dropping your calorie intake down too low, it's grumpy and sends signals telling you to over-consume food. Granny Smith turns up and sends you on a binge of everything you know you shouldn't be eating. This takes your overall weekly calorie intake way off the number needed for you to lose weight. In short, dropping your calorie intake too low has backfired. Instead, you need to find the sweet spot where you're in a calorie deficit, but it's not too low that Ghrelin gets grumpy and sends Granny Smith to come and feed you up.

To make weight loss straightforward, you must track your food intake to know how many calories you're consuming, what you're eating, and how you're eating.

TRACK YOUR FOOD INTAKE

This data will allow you to see what you need to change and what can stay as it is. This data clearly shows you whether you're going to lose weight, stay the same, or gain weight. We will use this data to look at ways you can improve your current eating habits. If there's one thing you must do to make your weight loss journey smooth, it's track your food intake. Doing this will allow you to see the numbers, removing any stress or uncertainty from the equation. Don't worry about what you're currently eating; focus on getting into the most crucial habit of logging everything you consume in MyFitnessPal. Take things one step at a time and focus on making just one change. Your smooth weight loss journey begins here by tracking your food intake.

Your To-Do List

1. If you don't already have it, download MyFitnessPal and set up your account.
2. Have a play with it and familiarise yourself with the app. Practice adding foods and navigating your way around to see the weekly calorie consumption, macronutrients, and meals.
3. Begin Tracking Your Food Intake.

5

GROW YOURSELF

Once upon a time, there was a weight loss coach. People bought his book to seek his help. In return, he would teach them the easy way to lose weight. One day, a person visited the weight loss coach for advice. "I have come to ask you to teach me about weight loss," the person said. After just a few minutes, it became apparent that the person was full of their own opinions and knowledge. They interrupted the coach repeatedly with their own stories and failed to listen to what the coach had to say. The coach calmly suggested that they should have a cup of Yorkshire tea. The coach began to pour his guest a cup, and it was soon filled, yet he kept pouring until the cup overflowed onto the table, the floor, and the person's lap. The person screamed, "Stop! The cup is full already. Can't you see?" "Exactly," the weight loss coach replied with a smile. "You are like this cup — so full of information that nothing more will fit in. Come back to me with an empty cup."

For clarification, this chat never happened, as I've reworded an old Chinese Zen saying, so don't go thinking I poured a cup of tea over a client's lap. I'd get cancelled at the drop of a hat. This story means that you can only take in a certain amount of information, just like the cup can only take in a certain amount of tea. You may feel like you know how to lose weight, but the truth is that you don't. Yes, you're experienced in losing weight, but you have read or been told vast information that has unfortunately filled your cup with water from a puddle in a park.

As we age, we fill our cups with our past experiences and knowledge. You purchased this book and put your trust in me. I will deliver, but when someone comes along and tells you that most of what you've been doing or know is useless, it is too easy to resort back to your existing beliefs. As it stands, your cup is full of beliefs such as weight loss is hard, requires sacrifice, salads, and diets are the only way you will lose weight. The cup must be emptied to allow yourself to believe and understand that weight loss can be easy and enjoyable. I don't wish for you to hold on to what you believe are the good parts and only empty the bad. Empty it all out.

If you don't empty your cup, you will not only keep hold of false beliefs but also suffer from information overload, which is a recipe for disaster. We only need a little key information; instead, we have loads of the stuff. Less is precise. Less is clear. Less is simple. Suppose you bring in more information and don't get rid of the other information you already know. In that case, it's just going to confuse you. The information you're bringing in will contradict the information you're holding. You often find that you retain information that doesn't help you at all, so I'm telling you to get rid of it. Most of it won't help you lose weight, and some will prevent you from losing weight. Don't drink the Kool-Aid.

In this book, I will provide information that will begin filling your cup up, chapter by chapter. Each chapter has been carefully created to provide the necessary information in the order that works. I'm mentioning this right now because this chapter contains three parts, which I will explain shortly. Each part is an essential part of growing yourself. Each requires space in your cup so you can absorb and retain the information I share. Please remove all the information you hold on to by emptying your cup. If you don't, you're just going to muddy the waters by drinking the muddy water.

Have you gotten rid of the clutter? Have you gotten rid of all the information you've learned about weight loss, healthy eating and dieting? Have you created space in your mind to begin absorbing all the vital information I will share in this chapter? You're ready to start if you have. If you still need to have a clear-out, then wait to move on until you have. Go for a walk and consider whether the information and methods you currently hold on to have helped or hindered you.

This may only seem minor to you right now; however, what I'm ensuring doesn't happen is you begin reading this content and thinking, "Yeah, but..." in the back of your mind. A person can't learn what they think they already know. When you talk, you are only repeating what you already know. But if you listen, you may learn something new. I need you to be committed to this process right now. You are in charge, in the driving seat, but to achieve your weight loss goal, you must flow through this book with a clear mind. Weight loss isn't as hard as you think, so don't begin with making it hard for yourself.

What does growing yourself mean?

Growing yourself may sound profound to some, and I suppose it is. We feel uncomfortable reflecting on our actions, discussing our thoughts and feelings, and working to improve our lives. The silly thing is, we shouldn't. Growing yourself is one empowering thing. When people set off to lose weight, they say to someone, "Tell me what to do, and I'll do it". They rely on someone else. Growing yourself is about discovering how to lose and control your weight in a way that will work specifically for you. To do this, you must understand the fundamentals of weight loss and why you do things. Knowing the reasoning behind things makes you more likely to stick to something. You're more likely to take the correct steps when you make the decisions. Tell me, and I forget. Teach me, and I remember. Involve me, and I learn.

Self-development is quite a hot topic these days. Don't worry; I'm not jumping on a trend or a fad. That's not how I work. Self-development is changing your mindset, outlook, and relationship with food and exercise. It's you becoming the best version of yourself. It means accountability, holding yourself responsible for your actions. When you slip up (because we all slip up on our weight loss journeys at some point), it allows you to put your hands up, admit what has happened, move on from it, get back on track, and continue your weight loss journey rather than dwelling on it and thinking negatively about the situation. Growing yourself is the acceptance that shit happens.

Growing yourself is having confidence in your ability. When you gain confidence in your ability, you feel empowered. When you feel empowered, you feel in complete control of your actions. And when you feel in complete control, you can lose weight and keep the weight off. You no longer feel food, negative feelings or a diet being in control. By growing yourself, it's you that's in control. Growing yourself isn't only about taking stock of your mindset and learning things; it's having fun too. We are led to believe that losing weight should be a punishment for the weight we have gained, which is nonsense. Just because you're losing weight, it doesn't have to be dull, restricted, or hard work. It shouldn't feel like a punishment or chore. It should be an enjoyable and uplifting journey. I want you to have fun on your weight loss journey because you're more likely to stick to things when you have fun, meaning you can fulfil your weight loss ambitions and stay at your target weight once you get there.

The three pillars of growing yourself

In Greek mythology, 'grasping the pillars' was a metaphor for reaching the ultimate in human achievement. For some, pillars marked the point at which one must turn back, acting as metaphorical limits. Growing yourself and reaching your full potential can seem scary for some and exciting for others. Going beyond the pillars is an unending quest for knowledge. The pillars become not a point of retreat but a gateway to the unknown. When you stand at the pillars, you must select one of two options - Turn back as you decide that you won't be able to achieve your goal, or step through the pillars on a quest for the knowledge that allows you to reach your weight loss goal. The three pillars you must walk through stand tall and make up the Grow Yourself chapter. Together, they create the fundamentals of your weight loss journey. Pillars distribute the weight of your journey and support you every step of the way. The knowledge shared within each pillar will stay with you and allow you to reach the ultimate in human achievement. Do you decide to turn back? Or are you ready to walk through?

The first pillar is Growing Your Mindset. Achieving anything in life begins with your mindset. It starts with you believing that you can achieve something. It begins with you thinking that you can do it. It's an overlooked part of your journey. Without it, you won't get very far. It's you deciding to walk through the pillars and live a life without limits. To break the glass ceiling the inner critic has placed above you. The second pillar is improving your eating

GROW YOURSELF

habits. Don't worry; I won't tell you to eat clean and cut out all your favourite foods. I'm also not going to tell you that you must consume mushrooms when you hate them. Simple and sound food advice is what you will get. The third pillar is being more active. I said active because it's about improving your activity levels. No need to worry—I won't tell you that you must spend your whole life in a gym or that you need to run a marathon any time soon. These are the three pillars of growing yourself you will be working through in this chapter. Let's get started!

PILLAR ONE
GROW YOUR MINDSET

Achieving anything in life starts with your mind. To achieve your weight loss goal, you must learn to look at things from a different perspective. The easiest way to explain this is by asking: Is the glass half full or half empty? I'm sure you've heard this said many times as it's a common expression; however, have you ever thought about the answer concerning your mind and behaviours? It represents your view on certain things. If you view the glass as half empty, you're pessimistic. If you consider the glass as half full, you're optimistic.

When setting off on your weight loss journey, you must always approach it with the view of the glass as half full—allowing you to think positively, look at what you already have, and consider what you could do to keep improving. Instead of beating yourself up about what you haven't achieved or don't have, you begin congratulating yourself on what you have achieved so far. You're happier and more content as you're grateful for what you have rather than being frustrated with what you have not. People tend to give up so fast because they look at how far they still have to go instead of how far they have come. Concentrate on putting one step forward, and never forget how far you've come. There's no such thing as starting from scratch. Every attempt to lose weight has been an opportunity to learn what you could do differently in the future.

Are you thinking, "Why do I need to grow my mindset?" Well, it all starts here. You may not believe it, but by the end of this pillar, you will understand your results will all depend on your mindset. If you think positively, you will have positive results. If you think negatively, you will have negative results. I've often experienced it from clients who have said things like— "I can't do it", "I'm a food addict", and "I'm destined to be this way for the rest of my life". No matter how knowledgeable or experienced I am as a weight loss coach, I can't help them get the desired results because they're mentally holding themselves back. Subconsciously protecting themselves from failing, something I will get to shortly. On the other hand, the clients who say things like—"I'm going to do this", "I'm going to change my life", and "I'm going to give this my all" go on to achieve some truly remarkable results.

We often take the power of our mind for granted, and we don't use its total capacity. It's the most powerful thing you possess, and it can accelerate your progress if you use it wisely. Use it positively, and you will achieve amazing things. Use it negatively; it will put you in a vicious circle of stress and worry. With a growth mindset, you can take on the world. It helps you take on problems and overcome any challenges or obstacles along the way. It enables you to find a way to get to where you want to be. There is always a solution to a problem. The most rewarding feeling is achieving the things you never thought possible. Breeding achievement is what growing your mindset is all about. "Right, I've achieved this. What else can I achieve?" runs through your head. You go from achieving one thing to looking for other parts of your lifestyle to improve. Before you know it, you've completed many things that complement one another—allowing you to control your weight and be more content with your life.

If you're thinking what a load of hippy twaddle, then think about what mindset you have and what it has done for you so far. I'm not asking you to begin a spiritual journey and find yourself in the mountains. I'm encouraging you to be more positive about yourself and your future. If you have a closed mentality and don't acquire a growth mindset, you will constantly be stuck where you are; I'm sure you don't want that. Without a growth mindset, you will avoid things challenging or taking you out of your comfort zone. Achieving new things seems scary rather than empowering. You stop at the pillars rather than going through the gateway to the unknown. You may put one foot past the pillar to see what it's like, but that only means you go into your weight loss journey half-hearted rather than fully committing to it.

The anticipation of failure and the fear of the unknown prevents you from achieving anything. You hit obstacles like a busy week or a plateau on your weight loss journey and instantly feel like you can't lose weight. Doubt and

GROW YOURSELF

worry start to take over in your mind. You're so busy worrying that you don't spend your time working out how to overcome the obstacle, causing you to give up because you believe you will be overweight for the rest of your life. You tell yourself you tried and feel weight loss is too hard to achieve, but deep down, you know you didn't give it a fair shot.

The feeling of weight loss being hard to achieve is due to exhaustion, a situation, and a lack of clarity. A growth mindset energises you rather than exhausts you by encouraging you to look at things optimistically. This newfound energy allows you to look at a situation through a different lens. You're sat on the train towards your destination rather than standing at the station watching it go by. The new outlook creates clarity, eliminating resistance and allowing you to lose weight smoothly. That's the power of your growth mindset. Have you been thinking about your current mindset? The easiest way to determine your current mindset is to agree or disagree with the following statements.

1. You are a certain kind of person, and nothing can change that.
2. No matter what kind of person you are, you can always change substantially.
3. You can do things differently, but the key parts of who you are can't be changed.
4. You can always change basic things about the kind of person you are.

Take a moment and consider whether you agree or disagree with these statements. If you agree with statements one and three, you're someone who has a fixed mindset. If you agree with statements two and four, you tend to have a growth mindset. If you agree with both one and two, I'm sorry; you're just confused. If you have a fixed mindset, weight loss can feel challenging. Don't worry, though, as you can change this.

There are four characteristics of a fixed mindset.

1. You believe your abilities are static, and you may get a little bit better or worse at specific skills.
2. Your abilities reflect how you're wired, and your behaviour is a good representation of your natural ability.
3. You avoid challenges. If you fail, you fear others will see your failure as an indication of your true ability and see you as a loser. Because of this belief, you don't face the challenge of losing weight.
4. You feel threatened by negative feedback. The critics say they are better than you, positioning themselves at a level of natural ability higher than yours.

You should never avoid trying to lose weight for fear of having others judge you. Only focus on yourself rather than worrying about what others think about you. It's your journey, and weight loss is something you want to achieve.

Most of the critics you hear are critics you've created in your mind. If you listen carefully, you will hear they aren't coming from other people. The inner critic is the most powerful thing holding you back from achieving your goals. It's scared of feedback so much, yet it's the one being negative. A fixed mindset is listening to the inner critic and allowing it to win. Avoiding challenges is another part of the inner critic dialogue and thought process. Nobody sees you as a failure if you get up on your own two feet and aspire to achieve your goal. You fear others will see your failure as an indication of your true ability; however, the inner critic within you sees this, not other people.

A fixed mindset prevents you from facing the challenge of losing weight. Due to the fear of negative feedback and avoidance of challenges, you believe your abilities are static because you haven't moved forward closer to your weight loss goal. A fixed mindset means you're a prisoner to your inner critic. It tells you that you may get a little bit better or worse at losing weight and that your abilities reflect how you're wired. It's okay to have a fixed mindset right now; however, you must flip the switch and gain a growth mindset to achieve your weight loss goal.

The next question I need to ask you is — Which step are you currently on? There are five steps to review and decide where you currently are. I want you to be honest with yourself when determining your current step rather than selecting the one you think you should be on.

Step One - I can't do it - The bottom step is where people say, "I can't do it?" It's the fixed mindset at its most powerful. The belief you can't do something means you won't have the energy, motivation, or time to take the next step. Unfortunately, many people are on this step, and it's the one that is the most difficult to get up from. People can be stuck on this step for their whole lives. If you believe you can't do something, you can't do it. It's that simple!

Step Two - I want to do it - A common place for people to begin is step two, where they say, I want to do it. Many people on this step say they want to lose weight but don't want to do it enough. Although they want to lose weight, they aren't willing to make the changes needed to achieve their weight loss goal. Changing parts of their lifestyle means stepping out of their comfort zone. They tend to move slowly and gradually up to step three, sometimes alternating between steps two and three. There is also another type of person who is on this step. It's the person who says, "I want to do it, and I will learn how". Once they've learnt how to lose weight in a way that works for them, they tend to skip step three and move straight to step four. If you're on this step, I'd like to think you're this type of person. After all, you've purchased a book and are ready to learn.

Step Three - I'll try to do it - "I'll try to do it" is the most tiring step to be on. It may sound productive; however, you're still stuck in the fixed mindset here. There's no conviction behind this statement. It's the step of the dilly-dally, dipping in and out of the actions needed to achieve your weight loss goal. You feel like you're taking action, yet instead, you're wasting precious energy that saps motivation and pulls you further back down to step one. You're so close yet so far. Instead of climbing up a ladder to steps four or five, you're sliding down a snake to step one. A common sign of people trying to lose weight is going on and off a diet or a sudden burst of exercise, then giving up shortly after. They're constantly sliding down the snake and climbing up the ladder, moving between steps two and three. It takes so much energy, and it's frustrating as they feel stuck and unable to achieve their weight loss goal. Eventually, they admit defeat and stop trying. You can't just say; I'll try to do it. You have to say I can do it.

Step Four - I can do it - This takes us up to step four, where I ultimately wish for you to be. "I can do it" is what people with a growth mindset say. If you believe you can achieve something, you will be able to achieve it. It provides the drive to your weight loss journey, so it becomes easy. Weight loss feels hard when you have a fixed mindset and easy when you have a growth mindset. Nothing phases you; you glide over obstacles and have fun along your journey. It may take time to switch from a fixed to a growth mindset; however, once you say to yourself, "I can do this", you will achieve your weight loss goal and have control of your weight in no time. Taking it back to the question: which step are you currently on?

Step Five - I did it - This step is where you achieve your weight loss goal and shout, "I did it". You make it to this step when a growth mindset and the two other pillars unite and make your weight loss journey easy. You need a growth mindset to make it to this step and reach your full potential. Can you instil a growth mindset in yourself? If you have already discovered that you have a growth mindset, that's amazing. But if you don't, then this is where you must listen and take the following information in.

There are three characteristics of a person with a growth mindset.

1. You believe your abilities are like muscles. People who have a growth mindset believe that abilities are like muscles. They can be built up with practice. With concerted effort, you can improve your eating habits, manage your cravings, or begin to enjoy exercise.
2. You accept more challenges despite the risk of failure. People with a growth mindset understand that failure is a part of life, and it's all down to how we react to these failures and improve ourselves. They seek out challenges in their life and enjoy the elements of overcoming them. The journey and the challenge are more rewarding than achieving their weight loss goal. They know that challenges strengthen and improve their characteristics.
3. You accept constructive criticism. By criticism, I mean reflecting on your previous actions and discovering how you can improve in the future rather than dwelling on the things that haven't worked for you. You want to learn and be better at

the things you currently need to improve. It's here where you begin to achieve some truly remarkable results.

Don't worry; it doesn't matter which mindset you currently have or which step you're on—You can change your perspective. The growth mindset can be taught and can change your life to create and sustain change, but you've got to be open to changing it. There will be some days when you can give 100%, and there will be many others when you won't. On the days when you only have 50%, give 50%. A fixed mindset sees 50% as not enough to give. A growth mindset sees that 50% is better than 0%. Every single action, no matter how big or small, is a step further down the road to weight loss.

You must act more like a coach and less like a scorekeeper. Scorekeepers solely focus on wins and losses. The wins are all that matter, and the losses are worthless. A coach is always looking for ways to help themselves or others be their best; even failures are opportunities for improvement. They've embraced failure as a means of growth. If you look at any successful sports team, they win and lose. However, what allows each team to win the league is learning from the losses to improve for the next fixture. This ensures they come out as the best team at the end of the season.

I provide you with the tools and structure to be your own coach. Throughout this book, I am your coach. However, once you've made it to the end, you will become your own coach and a successful one too. You will feel

GROW YOURSELF

empowered and in control of your weight loss journey and know what you need to do to improve as the years go by.

There are three things you must learn to adopt a growth mindset.

1. Real change, the change that sticks and creates sustainable results, is often three steps forward and two steps back.
2. Failure happens, some big and some small. You must understand that failure is a part of success.
3. If you persist with your weight loss journey, even if it looks like failure in the middle, it eventually emerges with a growing sense of positive momentum.

I've said it before, but I'll repeat it—You will fail. It may sound extreme, but the sooner you realise that failure is vital to any journey, the quicker you will achieve your weight loss goal. You've got to embrace it and learn from it. Sometimes, you will be tested, but this means you're stepping out of your comfort zone and either learning or improving. Failure and tests equal success; how you handle these tests makes you successful. A growth mindset will allow you to handle these tests easily and without stress. Finally, you will succeed. It may seem strange, but failure and learning from your own experiences are necessary to succeed. It's your job to learn and grow on your weight loss journey. To do this, you must grow yourself.

Your To-Do List

1. Discover which mindset you currently have. Look at the full statements to find out.
2. Discover what step you're currently on. Hopefully, it's step four.
3. Think about how you can grow your mindset and continue improving.

PILLAR TWO
EAT SMARTER

Pillar one provides the mindset needed to make weight loss easy and your life more content. Pillar two provides a way of eating that allows you to control your weight for the rest of your life. More often than not, people start by following a diet and then give up. This is because they have a fixed mindset, but it's also because they've been following a diet or way of eating that isn't sustainable for them. It's fixed, strict, and forceful. Do this, but don't do that. You can have an apple, but you can't have a Twix. Eat in the morning, but don't eat at night. The rules keep coming, but the results diminish. The more rules there are, the less likely you are to stick to something. This is why, in pillar two, I will provide clear guidelines for you to follow, but no set rules. A flexible way of eating is the long-term solution. At first, having so many choices may be scary or overwhelming. Still, you'll soon be happier when you realise how much freedom you have.

 If we strip food down, it is one of the necessities of life. We need food to survive. We can't avoid it and go cold turkey when losing weight. This means navigating long-term weight loss can be one of the most challenging journeys. I say long-term weight loss because short-term weight loss is pretty easy to navigate; drastically reduce your food intake, and you will see the weight fall off. This is why diets are so popular because they quickly give you the desired results. You've tried diets before and know they don't work long-term. A growth mindset prevents you from seeking instant gratification and encourages you to look at the bigger picture. It knows there's no point in restricting yourself for short-term weight loss, to do it all again in a couple of months. A growth mindset strives for a way that both the body and the mind are happy with, as it knows that when you are positive and content, everything feels more manageable.

To provide you with these feelings, I need to tell you right now that I'm not going to deny you of the foods you love. Food is fuel and all that jazz, but it's also there to enjoy. We celebrate around it by having a big Christmas dinner, a tasty cake on your birthday, or an anniversary meal with a loved one. You also catch up with friends over a couple of drinks and graze on popcorn or sweets when you go to the movies. Food brings people together, and you should never forget that. This is another reason why you must allow yourself to be flexible with your way of eating. Not every day or week is the same. It varies based on social situations, work commitments, and kids' activities. Think of all the social connections you will miss out on if you're strict with your eating. You must savour those moments, be thankful for what food brings to your soul, and understand that food doesn't just give you life; it gives you fulfilment too.

If I tell you to celebrate and go out with your friends, I'm sure you'll wonder where the problem lies. There has to be a villain in every story. When you walk into a supermarket, most of the food on the shelves is processed. They have taken out the 'good' stuff and replaced it with the 'bad' stuff. They have added salts, sugars, fats, and many other things I can't even pronounce. They have been stripped of fibre and nutrients. Foods such as rice, potatoes, and meats have been processed into crisps, deli meats, or cereals. It's not just the lack of nutrients and added salts, sugars, and fats that are a problem. You consume more calories from processed foods than unprocessed, even if you consume the same amount of calories from each. This is because processed foods have already been broken down, so the energy is readily available when it begins the digestion process.

When you consume unprocessed foods, the food has to be broken down within the body, meaning that the body has to use energy to do this. Do you remember the Thermic Effect of Food I mentioned in the understanding body weight chapter? The Thermic Effect of Food is responsible for 10% of a healthy adult's daily calorie burn. It's easier to gain weight when consuming processed foods, and it's easier to lose weight when consuming whole foods. Not all of the unprocessed food you consume will be broken down. Some pass through the body. This is why you shouldn't only calorie count. Instead, you need to look at the quality of your foods. Are they processed or unprocessed foods? It's all about calories absorbed and stored by the body, not just calories you put in your body.

I encourage you to consume most of your calories from unprocessed foods rather than processed. I'm not preventing you from consuming the foods you enjoy. Whole-natural foods are unprocessed and enjoyable too, and these foods don't just allow you to survive but thrive. Prioritise healthy carbohydrates, fats, proteins, vitamins, and minerals, and drink plenty of water. You will thrive if you consume something from each of these groups. If you do that, your body will be able to function correctly. You will have lots of energy, be healthy, and be able to lose weight and keep it off.

Whole-natural food isn't the same as eating clean. You can have a range of indulgent foods or meals by consuming whole-natural foods. It's a case of knowing how to make a birthday cake using as many natural products as possible rather than just whacking a candle in an avocado and downing a pint of water. This is why I'm encouraging you to follow the 80-20 principle, which tends to be the sweet spot for controlling your weight. Please ensure that 80% of your calorie intake comes from whole-natural foods, with the other 20% from the foods you enjoy. To confirm, it's 20% of your calorie intake from the foods you enjoy rather than 20% of the quantity of food you consume. People get caught out with that one as they associate calories with the size of something. A tiny chocolate brownie can pack a punch in terms of calories, so make sure you know I'm talking about 20% of your calorie intake. If you follow the 80-20 principle consistently, you'll be able to lose weight and keep it off because you're not actually on a diet. You're following a plan that works long-term because it's good for you. Yet, at the same time, it has space for the foods that you enjoy in moderation.

The final thing to say about the 80-20 principle is that it doesn't matter where you are right now. Remember, you're playing the long game. You may be at 50-50, which is fine. If you're there, aim to hit 60-40, then 70-30, until you hit the sweet spot of 80-20. This may take a few weeks or months, and that's ok. You will still lose weight if you track your calorie intake, so don't sweat and rush this. If you wanted to learn the guitar, you start with grade one and, over time, move on to grade two, until years go by and you're Jimi Hendrix. It takes time to master a skill, and the purpose of the 80-20 principle is to ensure you find a way of eating that provides the body with all the nutrients it needs whilst discovering a style of eating that will work long-term.

It's time to be smarter

Every person eats. Supermarkets have food. Restaurants cook for us. Cultures have their own flavours. There are so many ingredients, ways of cooking, and flavour combinations. My school used the six hours a year in food technology to make healthy, flavoursome, and cultured meals consisting of apple turnovers, fairy cakes, and the exotic sausage roll. The beige brigade was out in full force. Instead of teaching me about nutrition and how to cook, I made unhealthy foods that even the dog didn't want to eat when I got home. Not only was I denied the chance to learn about healthy foods and be taught the culinary skills of the world, I didn't stand a chance in The Great British Bake Off. How are we supposed to know how to eat healthy, balanced meals by rolling sausage meat in pre-made pastry sheets?

As we aren't taught about food, we are intimidated by words like quinoa, falafel, and mangetout. You might have been shown a food pyramid at some point, but do you know how to eat to live a healthy life and control your weight? The expectation of each person figuring it out is unrealistic. Just because we all eat and are adults, it doesn't mean we all turn into experts when we turn eighteen. We all earn and spend money, but that doesn't make us all good with it. Some make sensible decisions; others blow it all. Some people make smart food choices, and others make not-so-smart food choices. It's normal for us all to have different understandings of each topic. If you're not great with money, you don't need to read the Financial Times and become an accountant; you need to know your outgoings, why you make certain purchases, and what you could cut back on. If you've gained weight over time, you don't need to throw every food out the naughty cupboard and become a nutritionist; you need to know how to lose weight, understand what you're putting in your body, and decide what you could switch to allow weight loss to happen. You already know how to lose weight; it's now time to be smarter with your food choices.

I don't believe food is either good or bad, banished or allowed; this is why I encourage you to follow the 80-20 principle. I call unprocessed and nutritious foods smart food choices and processed and less nutritious foods not-so-smart food choices. Smart food choices make weight management easier, and not-so-smart food choices make weight management more difficult. You can lose weight if you only consume not-so-smart food choices if you like. It can be done as long as you consume fewer calories than your body requires. Please understand it will be more difficult; you will have to eat tiny portions and won't feel great. It's my purpose to show you that weight loss isn't as hard as you think, and for me to do this, I encourage you to make smart food choices not just on your weight loss journey but for the rest of your life.

Smart foods provide your body with the nutrients it needs to function correctly. Nutrients are compounds in foods that are essential to life and good health. As I just mentioned, they aren't essential to weight loss; however, they play a significant role in giving you the best chance to succeed on your weight loss journey and keep the weight off for good. They are the building blocks for repair and growth to keep you fresh and ready to take on the world. Nutrients are the substances needed to regulate over thirteen hundred chemical processes in the body. These include things like your metabolism and hormones, which play an important role in weight regulation. Smart foods decrease inflammation within the body, preventing illnesses and diseases. It allows your joints to function well, maintains mobility within the body, and allows you to move freely without any aches or pains.

It's not just your body that benefits from smart foods; they make you feel better too. You may have tried to lose weight before and felt tired and down; that's not the case if you have smart foods. They provide you with the energy needed to live a vibrant life. You will feel much better due to increased energy levels, improving your mood and allowing you to feel more positive about your weight loss journey. Generally, you can eat a greater quantity of smart food choices than not-so-smart food choices, meaning you can have more satisfying meals as they're not as calorific. You actually feel full even when losing weight, which is a game changer. At first, it may be challenging to get your head around as you're used to restrictions when losing weight, but you can eat more and still lose weight. Since you can eat more, you are happier to continue with this new way of eating as you will no longer feel like you're dieting or restricting yourself.

It's only fair to explain what happens if you aren't smart with your food choices. For starters, you may lose weight, you may not, but you will undoubtedly be pretty hungry. Losing weight with a majority of not-so-smart foods will show you that the total amount of food consumed each day is an amount that your five-year-old self would be fuming about. You believe that weight loss is all about eating less, so you cut your calorie intake but don't alter the foods you consume. It works for a short while, but you are always hungry and thinking of food because of this. The amount of food you've been consuming doesn't fill you up, causing you to consume foods you hadn't planned on eating. This bumps up your calorie intake because your body wants a greater quantity of food and nutrients, which prevents you from keeping off any weight you've lost. You're stuck in a world of yoyo dieting, spending your life either cutting food or re-feeding the body, which isn't generating sustainable results. Because of this, you think to yourself, "What's the point in trying?" and give up.

There is one more thing I need to outline. I've spoken about Leptin and Ghrelin being your hunger and fullness hormones, however, there's much more going on than this. There is a complex system of chemicals that send signals between your brain and your body. Your brain knows what it needs, but it can't tell you it needs a specific nutrient. What it can do is signal you're hungry. If the message gets across and you eat the type of food it wants, it will be happy and won't tell you to eat again. If it doesn't receive the food it wanted and receives a bag of crisps, it will tell you to eat again, leading to consuming more calories. You will have greater control of your calorie intake when consuming smart food choices. Your body will be satisfied with the food it receives, meaning fewer hunger signals and fewer calories consumed.

That's the weight loss side of things covered, but this is only a tiny part of why a diet full of not-so-smart foods is a not-so-good idea. They don't provide the body with what it wants and needs, preventing it from functioning as well as it could. This causes you to feel tired and irritable, lack focus, and hinders productivity and progression in all parts of life. Adding a lack of food to the equation causes you to be snappy, bad-tempered and impatient. Not-so-smart foods make us feel comforted, happy, and calm, but only while we eat them. Unfortunately, you're left with various negative feelings once these short-term positive feelings wane. Your body not functioning correctly is never good for you in the long-term, and I don't just mean in relation to weight loss. It can lead to the immune system being down, leaving you prone to various illnesses and diseases. Even if you don't wish to be healthier and are only bothered about losing weight, please think long-term about your health, emotions, and feelings. This is what someone with a growth mindset would do. There's no point in having the body you've dreamed of if you're ill. There is no point in having a slim physique if you don't have the energy to live life to the full. Take care of your body. It's the only place you have to live.

Tiny portions are the expectation of weight loss, but it isn't essential, so why do it? We constantly focus on cutting out foods or food groups, putting pressure on ourselves by saying we can't have certain foods. Yes, I've outlined the difference between smart and not-so-smart foods. I've explained that 80% of your calorie intake from smart foods and 20% from not-so-smart foods is the long-term sweet spot. I encourage people to eat, not diet, flipping the script and focusing on providing the body with what it needs. When I share the smart and not-so-smart foods with you, I want you to take the pressure off yourself and focus on including the smart foods. If you do this, the rest will take care of itself. Don't beat yourself up if most of your diet predominantly comprises not-so-smart foods.

Remember, as long as you're tracking your calorie intake, you will lose weight, allowing you to alter the quality of your food intake gradually. Don't strive for perfection on day one; focus on being better just a little bit each week.

Carbohydrates

Carbohydrates are classed as macronutrients along with Fats and Proteins. A macronutrient doesn't mean a massive baked bean; it means the body requires a large amount of that particular food group. If the body requires a large amount of them, it's absurd to heavily reduce or cut them out of the diet completely. Yet, most people on this planet are led to believe they should cut out carbs by numerous people in the industry without any real explanation. Carbohydrates are misunderstood, so it's important to understand what you're eating and whether it's good for you. The first misconception is that we should cut carbohydrates from the diet because they're bad for us.

The body uses carbohydrates to make glucose, the body's primary energy source. Glucose is a sugar that is immediately used by the body as energy. If the body receives more glucose than it needs for immediate energy, it is converted into glycogen, which is a reserve store of carbohydrates within the liver, skeletal muscles, and a small amount in your brain. Your body can only store up to 500g of glycogen before your stores are full, equating to 2000 calories worth of energy. Once these stores are full, the body begins to convert excess carbohydrates into fat so it can be stored in body fat cells instead. This is where people believe that carbohydrates can make you gain fat because, technically, they can be turned into body fat.

Another reason why people believe carbohydrates are bad for weight loss is because they are told that eating carbohydrates prevents the body from burning body fat as the body chooses to use the carbohydrates consumed instead. Don't get me wrong, the body loves some readily available energy in the form of glucose, but it isn't necessarily true. If you're in a calorie deficit, your body will have to burn body fat to make up the numbers. It doesn't matter if you consume carbs, don't consume carbs, or only eat doughnuts; your body will burn body fat if you're in a calorie deficit. Do carbohydrates prevent body fat from being lost? Absolutely not.

Another thing to mention concerning carbohydrates and fat loss is that carbohydrates enable fat metabolism, the process the body uses to convert body fat into energy for burning, which requires glycogen. As I mentioned earlier, glycogen is the reserve store of carbohydrates within the body. If there are no stored carbohydrates in the body, it will convert protein found in muscle tissue into glucose through a process called gluconeogenesis. This isn't a good idea as it's a lot of hard work for the body, and it's also burning muscle as energy. Muscle require lots of energy, which is good as it means your body needs more calories each day to maintain the muscle it has. Muscle also makes you look good and feel strong, so it's not wise to cut carbohydrates out of your diet to burn fat. It would actually be counterintuitive. Always keep in mind that fat burns in a carbohydrate flame. Carbohydrates, in some form, need to be present within the body for fat loss to occur without losing muscle simultaneously.

The final thing to say concerning carbohydrates and weight loss is that cutting carbohydrates from the diet will allow a significant drop in weight loss. Don't get your hopes up, though, as carbohydrate-cutting weight loss is temporary. The 500g of carbohydrates stored in the body as glycogen I mentioned earlier act as a massive sponge. Each gram of stored glycogen holds three to four grams of water. This means that you can hold 2kg of water within glycogen alone. If you cut carbohydrates from your diet, there is no glycogen to hold water, meaning a drop of 2kg or 4.4 pounds of body weight. People are impressed by the quick weight loss on a no or low-carbohydrate diet, but it's just water weight that's been lost, not an ounce of body fat. Once carbohydrates come back into the diet, glycogen stores are replenished, and the 2kg of body weight you lost instantly comes back because when a sponge gets wet, it gets heavier.

The reason why carbohydrates have a bad reputation is because of one word: sugar. It's a stigma that carbohydrates cannot shake off, no matter how hard they try, they're all tarred with the same brush. Sugar is the generic name for sweet-tasting soluble carbohydrates. There are simple sugars such as glucose, fructose, and galactose. There are also compound sugars such as sucrose, lactose, and maltose. Within the body, compound sugars are broken down into simple sugars. Sugars can be found naturally within plants such as corn, grains, and fruits. Corn is good for you, but a cheap source of sugar is corn syrup, which is not, and this is where the problem lies. We classify carbohydrates as having sugar within them and associate all sugars as bad. Still, the body uses glucose, which is sugar, as its primary source of energy, so we need it.

Food manufacturers have meddled with foods and turned perfectly healthy foods, such as corn, into unhealthy foods, such as corn syrup. If you source your sugar from natural whole foods, you will be fine, but if you source your sugar from manufactured processed foods, you will struggle with your weight. These products contain a ridiculous amount of added sugar, which makes us want more. Added sugar keeps their costs down, but our waistlines up. We are over-consuming sugar, which is why all carbohydrates are classed as bad in most people's eyes. A piece of fruit contains sugar, but it also contains a range of vitamins and minerals. A sweet potato contains sugar, but it also includes plenty of dietary fibre. Natural sources of sugar provide the body with other things that benefit the body, making them smart food choices. Added sugars and processed foods offer no benefit to the body, making them not-so-smart food choices.

Although all carbohydrates are converted to glucose for the body to use as energy, not all carbohydrates are created equally. Many carbohydrates, which I class as smart carbohydrates, provide the body with essential nutrients that allow the body to thrive. Your brain needs roughly 400 calories each day to function optimally, and its primary energy source is glucose, the sugars in carbohydrates. If you want to be able to focus, think and go about your day, then smart carbs are needed. There are also common features in people's diets that I classify as not-so-smart carbohydrates. These are high in added sugars, high in calories, and provide the body with no nutrients. They lead to weight gain along with being a cause of inflammation within the body, causing various illnesses and diseases such as diabetes, heart disease, and cancers.

Instead of cutting carbohydrates or ditching them altogether, you need to look at the type of carbohydrates you consume. Below, I have broken carbohydrates into three groups - Not-so-smart carbohydrates, which you should eat less often; not-as-smart carbohydrates, which you can eat sometimes; and smart carbohydrates, which you should eat more often. Don't worry about which carbohydrates make up most of your current intake; we will complete a task at the end of this pillar to improve it. For now, take a look at the carbohydrates within each category.

Not So Smart Carbohydrates - Eat Less Often

- Sugar
- Honey & Syrups
- Fried Potatoes
- Crisps
- Cereal Bars
- Crackers
- Foods with 10+ grams of added sugar

- Chocolate Bars
- Doughnuts
- Cookies
- Cakes
- Muffins
- Pastries
- Canned & Dried Fruit
- Fizzy Drinks
- Fruit Juices
- Flavoured Milk

Not As Smart Carbohydrates - Eat Sometimes

These foods contain some nutrients your body will benefit from but are less nutrient-dense than those in the Eat More section. You can eat these foods, but most of your carb intake should be based on the smart foods in the final section.

- White Rice
- Granola
- Couscous
- Instant or flavoured oats
- Milk
- Vegetable juices
- Flavoured yoghurt
- Pancakes and waffles
- Wholegrain crackers
- Oat-based granola bars
- Canned, dried, and pureed unsweetened fruit

- White bagels, bread, English muffins, pasta, and wraps

Smart Carbohydrates - Eat More Often

Eat more often are your smart food choices. These will keep you feeling fuller for longer. They contain plenty of fibre, which aids digestion, and they contain vitamins and minerals.

- Vegetables and lots of them
- Fruit
- Bean & Lentils
- Rolled Oats
- Buckwheat
- Quinoa
- Wholegrain, black and wild rice
- Millet
- Potatoes
- Plain non-Greek yoghurt
- Fresh and frozen fruit
- Corn
- Barley
- Sweet Potatoes
- Wholegrain bagels, bread, pasta, wraps and English muffins

Fats

Fats also have a bad reputation in relation to weight loss unless you've jumped on the Keto hype, of course, where you worship the ground they lard on. Just like carbohydrates, they're also macronutrients, meaning we need a large quantity of them, 0.5-1.0g per kg of body weight, to be precise. If our body needs many of them, why is everyone telling us they're bad for us? The reason behind this is that the word 'fat' is used to describe the food group, fat, and it's used to describe the storage of energy in the body, body fat. Although the word fat is used in both, it doesn't mean they are the same. Consuming fat doesn't make you fat.

In humans, excess dietary intake of carbohydrates and fat-rich foods, over and above what is needed for energy, leads to increased storage of body fat. This means if you go over your calorie intake, you will gain weight due to the storage of body fat. Most of this fat storage is a result of dietary fat due to the body choosing to use carbohydrates as energy first. Remember, the body's primary energy source is glucose, and it's readily available in carbohydrates rather than the body having to convert fat into glucose. Also, remember, fat burns in a carbohydrate flame, so just because excess dietary fat is stored as body fat due to the body choosing to use carbohydrates as energy instead, it doesn't mean you should cut your carbohydrate intake down. Instead, it would be best if you consume both carbohydrates and dietary fats in reasonable quantities that don't take you over your daily calorie requirements.

Another reason why fat has a bad reputation is because it's calorie-dense. One gram of dietary fat contains nine calories, whereas one gram of carbohydrates or protein contains four calories. Many people would see this as a reason to avoid consuming dietary fat, but you must understand that although all three are macronutrients, we don't need as much fat as carbohydrates or proteins. You don't need to worry about the exact amounts as, in general, when people consume a well-balanced diet, fat intake will naturally account for 15-20% of total dietary intake. An excessive restriction of fat intake to less than this amount often results in an unnecessary avoidance of a range of foods with otherwise valuable nutrient profiles. If you make smart food choices surrounding the types of fat in your diet, you don't need to specifically address your fat intake. Instead, you need to understand the role of dietary fat in supporting health and identify appropriate dietary sources of this macronutrient.

Fat is an essential component of a person's diet because it has several important roles in the body. The intake of dietary fat facilitates the absorption of fat-soluble vitamins and minerals, meaning that vitamins A, D, E, and K are only absorbed, transported and stored in the body if fat is present in the diet as it acts as the personal chauffeur to these VIPs. This is why it's always a good idea to drizzle some olive oil, sprinkle some cheese, or include some avocado or nuts on your salad. These fat-soluble vitamins improve eye health, skin quality, bone health, and much more. Fats form our brain and nervous system, allowing your brain to function correctly, therefore improving your memory, concentration levels, and thinking power. Finally, fats also help balance the various hormones within the body. These hormones help with muscle building and recovery, reducing inflammation and keeping your sex hormones going.

Not So Smart Fats - Eat Less Often

These are processed fats that contain little, if any, nutrients. Your job is to eat less of the foods in this section and gradually move towards consuming your fats from the eat sometimes and eat more often sections.

- Bacon
- Sausages
- Butter
- Margarine
- Processed Cheese
- Sunflower Oil
- Corn Oil
- Canola Oil
- Vegetable Oil
- Marinades and dressings with oils in this category
- Fat-rich foods with 10+ grams of added sugar
- Hydrogenated oils
- Trans fats
- Shortening

Not As Smart Fats - Eat Sometimes

These contain nutrients but less than the smart foods in the eat more often section. They are acceptable to eat, but they're just less beneficial than the eat more often foods.

- Virgin and light olive oil
- Pressed canola oil
- Sesame oil
- Flaxseed oil
- Coconut oil
- Coconut milk
- Peanut oil
- Regular peanut butter
- Dark chocolate
- Marinades and dressings with oils in this category
- Fish and algae oil
- Cream
- Cheese aged more than six months
- Flavoured nuts and nut butter
- Trail mix

Smart Fats - Eat More Often

It's your job to consume the smart fats from this section. We want better fats, not fewer fats. These smart fats are the ones that your body will benefit from.

- Extra virgin olive oil
- Walnut oil
- Avocado and avocado oil
- Marinades and dressings with oil in this category, including pesto
- Cheese aged less than six months
- Egg yolks
- Seeds - Chia, flax, hemp, pumpkin, sesame

- Cashews
- Pistachios, Almonds, Pecans, Peanuts
- Brazil nuts
- Natural nut butter from this category
- Olives
- Fresh, unprocessed coconut

Protein

Whilst fats and carbohydrates battle it out for the crown of apparent villain, protein is put on a pedestal. It's so powerful you can now place 'with protein' on unhealthy packaging, and people will buy it. No matter what food it is, if it's with protein, it's getting into the body under the false pretence that it's healthy. Snickers with protein, healthy or is it still a chocolate bar? Weetabix with protein, less or more protein than the original ones? Brands have jumped on the rise in popularity and labelled protein on everything. Fridge raiders have the slogan, powered by protein, on the packaging. Yes, chicken has protein in it, but processed meats like fridge raiders aren't the best source of protein. Eat a chicken breast instead.

Protein has become the champion macronutrient for many reasons. Although the body can technically convert protein to body fat, the fact of the matter is that it can't really be bothered to. Just like a teenager tidying their room, it's too much effort. The body likes things to be easy, so it will always choose to store excess dietary fat as body fat, store excess carbohydrates as glycogen, and simply excrete excess proteins. This is why protein seems untouchable, as the body will never store it as body fat. People need to understand that just because excess protein doesn't directly end up stored as body fat, it will indirectly lead to the storage of body fat if you exceed your daily calorie intake. Remember that you will gain weight whenever you over-consume energy in the form of calories, no matter what it is. Increasing your daily protein intake is a good idea, as most people don't consume sufficient daily amounts. However, just like any food, eating an uncapped quantity is not a good idea.

Another reason why protein is seen as a Demigod is its ability to help you control your weight by keeping you fuller for longer than other macronutrients. Although protein only contains four calories per gram, the same as carbohydrates and five calories less than fat, those same calories take longer to be digested. Protein also reduces your hunger hormone Ghrelin, controlling your appetite and making you feel fuller for longer. If you want to eat less, eating more protein makes sense. If you're a late-night snacker or daily grazer, protein may be just what you need. Cravings can be tough to control, so it's always a good idea to prevent them from occurring. This way, you don't have to control them. As protein keeps you feeling fuller for longer and controls your appetite, you suppress the urge to search in the cupboards for a treat or two. Is it advisable to consume sufficient protein if you're looking to control your appetite and cravings? Absolutely!

You now see how protein affects your appetite and weight control, but that's only the beginning. Earlier in this book, I explained to you that the body weight you aim to lose is body fat. Unfortunately, people strive for big numbers on the scales and don't think about the type of weight they are losing. When they do this, they lose some fat, water and muscle. Muscles are important because they require a lot of calories to maintain themselves, meaning that your metabolism will be higher and your daily calorie intake can be higher, too. The more muscle you have, the more calories your body requires. This is good when maintaining weight as it means you have a buffer to play with, as your body will require more calories than somebody with less muscle. It's also good to keep the muscle mass you've got when losing weight, as the less muscle mass you have, the fewer calories you will have to consume each day, making fat loss challenging to stick to. Muscle helps with weight control and weight loss due to the demands of this energy-rich tissue.

If you want to lose weight, your goal is to look good. If that's the case, it's not just weight loss that will help. Weight loss makes you slimmer in all areas of the body, which may sound good to you, but you have to think about what that means. If you lose weight without keeping or gaining muscle, then your size will decrease; however, you will be left with excess skin that has nothing to shape itself around. The body you've always dreamed of will never appear unless you keep or increase your muscle mass, which is another reason why protein is so popular these days. Elevated daily protein intake in the range of 2.3 grams per kilogram of body weight has been shown to maintain muscle mass in the face of a calorie deficit. This is why increasing your habitual protein intake may be beneficial when losing weight. Protein maintains muscle by providing the muscle with what it needs to regenerate. Think of protein as the sun to a plant and carbohydrates as the water. If you consume the two and do some resistance training, you will bloom into a beautiful flower. The body you've always dreamed of will become a reality.

It's not just muscle that benefits from protein intake. Consuming smart proteins helps you build, maintain, and replace the tissues in your body. These are your muscles, organs, and immune system. Proteins are essential for movements generated by muscle contractions. Muscle contractions are possible thanks to the action of the proteins actin and myosin, which interact to produce mechanical force within skeletal muscles. Antibodies produced by the immune system are also proteins which can recognise and neutralise microorganisms (pathogens) that may cause disease. The antibodies degrade and destroy the foreign substances in the body to maintain good health. Oxygen, required for aerobic metabolism, is transported around the body by a protein called haemoglobin. Fatty acids, the building blocks of fat in our bodies and in the food we eat, are transported around the body by a protein called albumin. The transport of many molecules, such as glucose, calcium, sodium, and potassium, in and out of cells relies on protein.

I could be here all day discussing many other benefits of consuming smart proteins and their roles. Hopefully, you can see what the hype is all about by now, but this doesn't mean you need to begin chugging protein shakes. You need to know your current protein intake by looking in

MyFitnessPal. If you find it's lower than 1g per kilogram of your current body weight, aim to increase your smart protein intake to around 2g per kilogram. This will ensure you maintain the muscle mass you currently have when losing body fat.

Not So Smart Proteins - Eat Less Often

- Fried meats
- Chicken fingers, nuggets, and wings
- High-fat ground meat
- High-fat sausages
- Processed soy products
- Processed deli meats
- Protein bars
- Pepperoni sticks
- High mercury fish

Not As Smart Proteins - Eat Sometimes

- Medium lean meats
- Uncultured cottage cheese
- Edamame beans
- Tofu
- Poultry sausages
- Minimally processed lean deli meats
- Protein powders
- Beef jerky

Smart Proteins - Eat More Often

- Eggs and egg whites
- Fish
- Shellfish
- Chicken
- Duck breast and thighs
- Turkey
- Lean beef
- Bison
- Lamb
- Pork
- Wild Game
- Kangaroo, goat, camel, crocodile
- Plain greek yoghurt
- Cultured cottage cheese
- Tempeh
- Lentils and beans

Vitamins and Minerals

If you aim to consume smart carbohydrates, fats, and proteins within your daily calorie requirements, you're not only going to lose weight, but you'll keep the weight off. Transitioning to smart foods, most of the time, creates a new way of eating that you and your body will be happy with. I'm finishing this pillar with something that gets overlooked, as you don't technically need them to lose weight. They perform hundreds of essential roles within the body, and they are vitamins and minerals. Vitamins and minerals are generally referred to as fruits and vegetables but are in many other things too. You will find them in all smart fats, carbohydrates, and proteins. We are told to eat five a day, with some campaigning to eat ten a day, yet most people don't. Although they're not essential to your weight loss goal, I'm hoping I could sway you to consume more of them.

Vitamins and minerals are micronutrients, meaning you don't need much of each. What we do need is a variety of them to allow our bodies to function correctly. There are thirteen essential vitamins that your body needs. These are vitamins A, B, C, D, E, and K, which only equates to six. This is because eight of the thirteen essential vitamins come from the B group. Eight B vitamins plus A, C, D, E, and K equals thirteen. In addition to this, your body also requires fifteen essential minerals, such as calcium, iron, and potassium. Overall, that's twenty-eight essential vitamins and minerals, so let's briefly go over what they do.

Vitamins and minerals are essential for good health and longevity, working in symphony to grow, heal, repair and maintain your body's cells, organs, systems and skeleton. They are needed to protect you from diseases, maintain bone health, aid digestion, help ferry oxygen around the body and play a key role in your metabolism. They protect your vision and eye health, which is why the saying carrots let you see in the dark is even a thing. In terms of image, they keep your skin looking fresh, your hair smooth, and your nails strong. The list could go on, but I'm sure you understand. I haven't covered the essential minerals or gone into greater detail about each of the eight B vitamins. This is because it's my job to make things easy for you and ensure you don't sweat the small stuff.

The simplest way to get everything you need is to eat food from each colour group - Red, Green, Yellow/Orange, Blue/Purple, and White, where eating five portions of fruit and vegetables a day logically comes from. I'm sure you've heard people tell you to eat the rainbow, this is why. Each colour provides something different; therefore, eating the rainbow will ensure your body receives all the vitamins and minerals it needs. The primary goal is to eat the rainbow, but if you can, aim to eat as many different foods from each colour. The greater the range, the better, which is why some people encourage others to eat ten portions of fruit and vegetables per day. Ideally, you would consume food from each colour each day, but sometimes you don't feel like it, and that's fine. Aim to include as many of them as possible. Let's take a look at the foods in each colour.

Reds

- Tomatoes
- Cranberries
- Cherries
- Strawberries
- Raspberries
- Grapefruit
- Watermelon

- Pomegranates
- Red Cabbage
- Papaya
- Chillis
- Chilli Powder

Greens

- Spinach
- Kale
- Pepper
- Cabbage
- Brocolli
- Green peas
- Green beans
- Brussel Sprouts
- Parsley
- Limes
- Green Tea

Yellow & Oranges

- Oranges
- Lemons
- Mango
- Pineapple
- Peaches
- Pumpkin
- Carrots
- Butternut Squash

- Sweet Potato
- Ginger
- Turmeric

Blue & Purples

- Blueberries
- Blackberries
- Grapes
- Aubergine
- Beetroot
- Prunes
- Cacao Powder
- Red Wine

Whites

- Coconut
- Apples
- Onions
- Parsnips
- Mushrooms
- Garlic
- Bananas
- Cauliflower

You may find that you consume a reasonable amount of food from one colour but not the others. Aim to consume at least one food from each colour each day. It's the final piece to the pillar of improving your eating habits. By now, you should see that weight loss isn't about cutting foods; it's about providing the body with better food choices. If you focus on what to eat, rather than what not, you will view weight loss and weight management in a completely different way. You look at foods that benefit the body and make you feel great, and you look at others that subtract value from your body. You don't feel full or well nourished when you consume not-so-smart food choices, yet you do when you consume smart food choices. At the same time, you haven't banned anything. You no longer believe in "good" or "bad" foods, so on special occasions, you enjoy a dessert and don't feel guilty. Associating foods as either good or bad creates a negative relationship with food. A negative mindset creates negative eating habits; we don't want that. That's why I've categorised each food group as eat more often, eat sometimes or eat less often. Just because you've eaten something from the eat less often column, it's not the end of the world. Today, think about how you can improve your eating habits by a small amount. You don't need to change everything all at once; just ask yourself: Do the foods I currently eat add value to my body?

Your To-Do List

1. Look at your current weekly food intake on MyFitnessPal and place each food you've consumed into one of the three columns. This will allow you to see whether the foods you consume

are mainly from the eat more often, eat sometimes, or eat less often column.
2. Then, it's your mission to gradually move as much of your diet to the eat more often column as possible. To do this, you do a task I call stick, switch, and ditch. In this task, you look at your current food intake and decide which foods you're keeping, which foods you're switching, and which foods you're ditching.
3. Then, task three is all about fruits and vegetables. It's important to get some variety in each day, so your task is to discover which colours you're missing out on regularly and then decide which foods from that colour you could include in your diet.

PILLAR THREE
BE MORE ACTIVE

A question I always get asked is, "Do I need to exercise to lose weight?" This is why I am answering this question for you right now. You don't need to exercise to lose weight, and I'm certainly not going to tell you that it's compulsory. It's your weight loss journey and life, so you can do as you please. I just thought I'd inform you that, in case you were shaking at the thought, you may have to join a gym. You can relax now. To lose weight, you must be in a calorie deficit and allow your body to function correctly by consuming a balanced diet. This means you don't need to exercise to lose weight, but you should realise that it will help in many ways. I've used the word exercise as that's what people are familiar with; however, being more active is more than a visit to a gym; it's a lifestyle.

If you don't need to exercise to lose weight, then why should you do it? When losing weight, you must ensure you're in a calorie deficit. This means you're consuming fewer calories than your body is burning off. You can be in a calorie deficit by consuming fewer calories by decreasing your food intake or by increasing your calorie output by being more active. Increasing your calorie output means you won't need to drop your food intake as much. The sweet spot is a calorie deficit of 500-700 calories per day. You can consume 250-350 calories less and burn off 250-350 calories through exercise. Consume 500-700 calories less and not burn any extra calories. You could also consume maintenance calories and burn 500-700 calories through exercise. The choice is yours. All you need to do is be in a calorie deficit. There will be some days when you wish to have a larger meal or are going out for food. As this will increase your calorie intake, it would be sensible to exercise on this day. There will be other days when you don't have the time to exercise. Due to this, it would be sensible to reduce your calorie intake by 500-700 calories.

	Mon	Tue	Wed	Thurs	Fri	Sat	Sun	Total
Target	1500	1500	1500	1500	1500	1500	1500	10500
Food (Calories In)	1500	1700	1600	1900	1500	2000	2000	12450
Exercise (Calories Out)	0	250	100	500	0	600	200	1900
Total	1500	1450	1500	1400	1500	1400	1800	10550

Above is a table showing the weekly calorie intake through food and the weekly calorie output through an individual's exercise. A busy day at work meant they couldn't exercise on Monday, so they went into a calorie deficit through food alone. Tuesday's evening meal consisted of red meat, which contains more calories than white meat. For this reason, they ensured they did a brisk walk after dinner with their partner. Wednesday was a calorie deficit mainly caused by food intake. They did some squats and press-ups in the evening. Thursday consisted of an exercise class where they burnt 500 calories, allowing them to consume a larger-than-usual lunch and dinner. Their calorie deficit was achieved through exercise alone. Friday was a quiet one socially, and they wanted an evening on the sofa, so they ensured they were in a calorie deficit through food intake alone. Saturday morning consisted of a park run where they burnt 600 calories. This meant they could go out with friends, consume 2000 calories, and still lose weight. Sunday consisted of a Sunday Roast, which took them to 2000 calories for the day. They did some squats, press-ups, lunges, and sit-ups in the morning and burnt 200 calories. They exceeded their target by 300 calories; however, when looking at their weekly total, they saw they were on target to lose weight this week.

The above example shows that you can be in a calorie deficit through food intake, exercise output, or a combination of the two. The beauty of knowing how to lose weight is that you can decide your own strategy to be in a calorie deficit. Exercise gives you options. If you try to lose weight through food intake alone, there is no flexibility in how many calories you can consume to lose weight. As the example outlines, you don't have to join a gym or run 5km. You can increase your calorie output by doing bodyweight exercises, going for a long walk with your family, taking the stairs, or swimming. The choice is yours.

Building lean muscle mass through resistance training can increase your resting metabolic rate, making it easier to control your weight. Muscle requires lots of energy to maintain, so you can consume more calories each day and not gain weight. Dwayne "The Rock" Johnson consumes six to eight thousand calories per day, and he looks in excellent physical condition. This is due to his muscle mass requiring lots of calories. If he didn't have this amount of muscle mass, then he would be morbidly obese. Do you smell what the rock is cooking? Weight training is one of the best ways of controlling your body weight in the long term. Don't go doing sit-ups and bicep curls. The best way to build muscle is to train the biggest muscles in the body. These are your legs, back, chest, and shoulders. Can you implement any of the following exercises into your weekly routine?

Bodyweight exercises - Squats, Lunges, Press Ups
Free weight exercises - Squats, Deadlift, Straight Leg Deadlift, Single Arm Row, Chest Press, Shoulder Press
Resistance Machine exercises - Leg Press, Chest Press, Lat Pulldown, Seated Row, Shoulder Press

When building muscle, you need to lift a weight that challenges you. Initially, this could be your body weight, but then you will need to gradually increase the load to build muscle as you get stronger. Don't be put off lifting heavy weights; they're good for you in many ways. Seek help from a qualified professional to ensure you're doing them safely and effectively. I've mentioned weight training first because it's the first type of exercise you should implement into your weekly routine. Weight loss through a calorie deficit will help you lose weight, but weight training will help you transform your body shape. Although one of the key reasons for weight training is to help you keep control of your weight once you achieve your weight loss goal, it's always best to begin lifting weights at the beginning of your weight loss journey. Doing it this way allows you to maintain good shape. It takes time to build muscle, so the earlier you start, the better. You won't have the misshapen middle of your weight loss journey where you've lost half of your weight target but don't feel great when you look in the mirror. Each month will be a transformation you're proud of.

Increasing your muscle mass through weight training allows you to burn calories even when you aren't doing anything due to muscles requiring plenty of energy. Another form of exercise, known as interval training, allows you to burn additional calories when sitting on the sofa. It is a high-intensity exercise style; however, if you can do it, it's the most efficient way of exercising. First, you don't need to do it for too long. A twenty-minute session consisting of one minute at a high intensity followed by one minute of rest would be sufficient. Second, this high-intensity session elevates oxygen consumption and metabolism, known as excess post-exercise oxygen consumption (EPOC for short). EPOC is the process that helps restore your body to its pre-exercise state. Due to the high intensity of your exercise session, your metabolism continues increasing for 24-48 hours after you've finished exercising, meaning a more significant calorie burn even when you're not doing anything.

Weight and interval training are by far the most efficient and effective ways of burning additional calories and controlling your body weight, fitting into busy schedules. Doing two twenty-minute interval sessions and two weight training sessions per week is the ideal volume of work and rest. Your body takes time to recover to its pre-exercise state, so every other day would be recommended for exercise as you allocate a day of rest and recovery in between. These exercise types may not be for you. It's your life and your weight loss journey. There are other forms of exercise that you may find are more suitable for you and your lifestyle.

Exercise doesn't have to be hundred-mile-an-hour interval sessions; it can be continuous exercise sessions such as going for a run, a walk in the countryside, swimming at the leisure centre, cycling to work, playing a sport, or dancing in your living room like nobody is watching. Exercise is anything that gets your heart rate up. An exercise session is only effective if you do it, so if you don't feel comfortable doing weight training or interval training, then you aren't going to stick to it. The best place to begin fitting exercise into your weekly routine is to find something you're happy doing. Yes, some are more effective and efficient than others, but something is better than nothing.

Nothing means you won't feel energised; instead, you will feel tired and sluggish. This feeling forces you to make not-so-smart food choices and search for instant energy-boosting food such as sugary treats. Calorie intake remains high, yet metabolism remains slow, meaning your calorie input vs output equation is incorrect. Nothing is the butterfly effect of remaining tired, leading to a diet consisting mainly of not-so-smart food choices, causing you to have a slow metabolism and over-consume calories, meaning being unable to lose weight. The butterfly blinks and doesn't flap its wings, and all of this happens. Suppose the butterfly flaps its wings. In that case, you increase your energy levels, making you feel amazing, which influences you to provide the body with smart food choices, boosting your metabolism and allowing you to lose weight easily. You don't have to become a Marine or Paula Ratcliffe; you need to flap your wings and let the butterfly effect do its thing.

Exercise sets the butterfly effect in motion; when this happens, you benefit in many ways. Not only does it aid in weight loss and weight control, it improves your health. By exercising, you strengthen your immune system, meaning a reduction in illnesses and the ability to fight disease. It strengthens your muscles, bones and joints, which helps you look good, feel strong, improve posture, and reduce the risk of osteoporosis. Exercising enables you to de-stress and sleep better, which is always beneficial if you eat when stressed. The growth mindset strengthens as you gradually improve your ability to do things you didn't believe were possible. You are proud of yourself, feel strong and confident, and look a million dollars. Exercise is a celebration of what the body can do and makes your lazy days feel much more rewarding.

To finish this pillar and go full circle, I would like to ask you two questions. The first is, "Do you need to exercise to lose weight?". As you can see, it's not as straightforward as yes or no, is it? If you simplify the answer, the answer is no; you technically don't need to exercise to lose weight. However, exercise helps you lose and control your weight, among many other things. The second question is, "Are you going to exercise to lose weight?". Now that you have been provided with the information shared in this pillar, I'd like to know if you have decided to implement some form of exercise into your weekly routine. It's your weight loss journey, meaning you decide what you want to do. That's the beauty of this book, you decide.

Some will still say no, they're not going to exercise to lose weight; others will say it's a must. Some will go for the high-intensity sessions, and others may be more active by walking daily. People are often put off doing exercise due to being told to do it all the time and do lots of it. You can do ten minutes a day, twenty-minute sessions three times per week, or two one-hour sessions per week. You also don't need a workout plan. A workout plan is just a plan created by somebody else. It has their preferences and ideologies in mind. Instead, the long-term plan needs to be created by you, and I will help you discover a way of being more active that works for you later on in this book. For now, understand the benefits of being more active. When you add it to your growth mindset and be smarter with your food choices, your excess weight will easily fall off.

Your To-Do List

1. Map out your day to see how active you are on a typical day.
2. Look at parts of your day where you could move more.
3. Decide what activities you could do at the times when you could move more.

6

BRIGHT SPOTS

When we have the option of looking at the positive or negative side of things, we tend to draw our attention to the negative. Right now, you have many thoughts and feelings about yourself. How many positive things will you say about yourself compared to how many negative? I'm a Manchester United fan, and I can tell you plenty of negative things about the club compared to the positive. It's naturally within us to focus on the negative side of things, which is why it's ok for us to do it. There's not much we can blame ourselves for when something is a natural response. Even in that previous sentence, I'm searching for blame or other negative thoughts or feelings. This doesn't mean I'm a negative person. This means that when assessing or evaluating anything, we naturally begin with the negative. If you find yourself doing this, you must notice and name it. Identify that you're starting with the negative, stop yourself and aim to begin with the positives.

These positives are known as your bright spots and are simply things you're already doing well in your life. In the Grow Yourself chapter, you were made aware that you must first gain a growth mindset. Looking at the positive instead of the negative is precisely that. Bright spots are the best hope for directing the rider when trying to bring about change. When you begin with your bright spots, everything looks much more straightforward, and the task is easier to achieve. If you don't find your bright spots, the rider procrastinates, so no action is taken. It's a form of protection as everything seems overwhelming. The rider doesn't know how to act, and instead of taking positive and rational steps, they allow negative emotions to decide what to do and where to go. The elephant controls your journey rather than the rider, causing you to head in the wrong direction and end up in a circle of stress and worry, which is hard to escape.

You now know that a bright spot is something you already have going well for you, but what are you supposed to do with it? It's pretty simple. All you have to do is investigate why it's already going well for you and then try to clone this success to help you on your weight loss journey. A bright spot could be a trait such as being organised at work. You could study it to discover how you could be organised with your meals or exercise routine. A bright spot is anything that you already do well. A lot of the time, we act in different ways in certain situations. We give positive advice to others yet are critical of ourselves. We are organised at work, but can't find the discipline to be organised with our meals. We take our kids to activities but don't take ourselves to the gym. This is why it's important to look at all aspects of your life to discover your bright spots.

When setting off on your weight loss journey, people tend to attack it in an unsustainable way. Their rational and emotional thinking battle it out for a couple of weeks until the elephant wins. This is why people say they lack the willpower to succeed on their weight loss journey. What they are trying to do is fight a losing battle. There will only ever be one winner, and it's certainly not their fault. If the elephant and the rider ever fight, the elephant will always win. You can't fight it; you must factor it in instead. Bright spots allow you to follow the road of least resistance. If there is ever any resistance, the elephant won't like it. This is why you need to clone what's already going well. If you ever have two options you can make, one seems simple and the other more complex, you must get into the habit of picking the easier one every single time.

We all have the same amount of energy. It's up to us as individuals to decide whether we channel this energy on the negative, which will slow things down, decrease motivation and create more negative feelings; or focus on the positive, which will speed things up, increase motivation and create more positive feelings. There will always be things you are doing well and others you aren't. Ask yourself, "What would your weight loss journey look like if it was easy?". This is one of the most important questions to ask yourself. We all have our own ideas of what easy looks like; sometimes, we don't even think about these things. Instead, we spend all of our time thinking about how hard it is to achieve something. We are often told that weight loss requires sacrifice, hard work, and restriction. But this doesn't have to be the case. Easy is replicating the positives for more positives. Focusing on your bright spots makes your weight loss journey effortless.

Before I help you discover your bright spots, I encourage you not to let this happen. You start off well by cloning your bright spots but are drawn to changing the negatives. It's easy to follow the road of least resistance by cloning your bright spots. It's a rational decision based on the rider. However, the elephant feels it should be doing more. Our emotions feel like we are slacking and should be sacrificing things, sparking hatred towards our own journey, like we are supposed to hate every part of the weight loss process. It doesn't make sense at all, but that's how we are programmed. If you ever find yourself leaving the road of least resistance and begin tinkering with some negatives. You need to notice and name it. Never take a foot off this road and start charging through thorny bushes. You may think this all sounds like it never happens, but trust me, it does. When things are easy, instead of enjoying the journey, we ask ourselves what more we could do. But you don't need to do anything. Just kick back and enjoy the ride.

It's now time for you to begin to discover your bright spots. What are you doing well, and how are you succeeding in that particular part of your life? Once you've learnt and discovered how you are succeeding in that part of your life, you can clone these actions and bring them into your weight loss journey, giving you the best chance of success. Instead of starting your weight loss journey with force and negativity, you begin with a positive mindset because everything looks effortless.

What are you doing well at work?

- Are you turning up on time?
- Are you organised with your workload?
- Are you positive and driven to succeed?
- Are you able to solve problems by finding solutions?

If you turn up on time to work, you have good time management. You can manage your time and tasks outside of work if you are organised with your workload. If you're positive and driven to succeed in your career, you can be positive and driven to succeed on your weight loss journey. If you can solve problems by finding solutions at work, you can overcome any barriers that may get in your way. How and why are you successful with these bright spots? How can you clone them to make yourself more organised, positive, and driven to succeed on your weight loss journey?

What are you doing while at home?

- Are you cooking most of your meals?
- Are you eating at the table without distractions?
- Are you caring towards your family?

If you're cooking most of your meals, that's brilliant. This is a big bright spot, as you know what goes into every meal. If you're eating at the table without distractions and can focus on eating slowly and mindfully, that's a bright spot, as it plays a big part in weight loss and controlling your food intake. If you care about your family, you can learn to be caring towards yourself rather than negatively thinking of yourself; that is a bright spot too.

What are you doing well in health?

- Are you exercising sometimes?
- Are you eating nutritious meals on certain days?
- Are you more active at certain times of the week?

If you're exercising sometimes, that's great, as you already do something your health will benefit from. If you're eating nutritious meals on certain days, that takes out a meal that isn't nutritious during the week. If you are more active at certain times of the week, think about how to implement this into other days of the week.

What can you learn from this? - Once you've identified your bright spots, it's time to investigate why they are bright spots. Please think about what you can learn from them and how you can replicate these positive actions. To get thinking, ask yourself the following three questions to commence the investigation.

Which days of the week are better? - Within each week, you will find that certain days are better than others. You need to find and discover what you are doing well on these days to allow you to replicate them on those that aren't going as well.

What actions are better? - Actions get results no matter what area of your life they are in. Suppose you are organised with your family time; how could you be organised at meal times? Can you allocate time to sit down and eat your meal without distractions or set aside some time to do a ten-minute workout?

When is your mentality better? - You will find that your mentality is better in some areas of your life than others. Suppose you're motivated to succeed at work. How could you replicate this so you're motivated to succeed on your weight loss journey? If you encourage your kids to do their homework, then how can you encourage yourself to do some form of exercise?

Once you have discovered what you're doing well and have thought about what you can learn from this, you need to think about how to clone this success. The point of your bright spots is to clone them so your progress gets smoother. You are replicating them to make change easier. I've provided you with three key questions to ask yourself about your bright spots, but this doesn't mean they are the only questions you should ask. Dig as much as you can into these already successful habits to discover how they can help make your weight loss journey easier. If there are bright spots directly related to your eating habits or exercise routine, such as cooking all meals at home, ask yourself how you can get even better at them.

BRIGHT SPOTS

A bright spot such as this is a golden nugget. This is the best place to start.

Before you clone any bright spot currently outside your eating habits or exercise routine, you must ask yourself whether cloning each particular bright spot will make your weight loss journey easier, to think more positively and begin on the front foot. The whole idea of discovering and cloning your bright spots is to ensure your journey is as smooth and straightforward as possible. To do this, you must think of the easy changes to make rather than the hard ones, as it's easier to clone them than create new ones that will be more challenging. Remember, you must follow the road of least resistance, which is why the easiest and most effective bright spots are the ones to clone first. Some bright spots are worth cloning, and others aren't, so before you clone one, always ask yourself - Will cloning this bright spot allow me to lose weight easily?

We are coming to the close of this chapter, which has been relatively short and sweet compared to others. This doesn't mean it isn't as important; it's just based on one thing. I encourage you to take the time to discover your bright spots, investigate them, and clone them. This is often overlooked as it seems too simple to be true. The elephant believes it should focus on the negative aspects. Still, the rider knows that to get where you need to be, you must follow the road of least resistance by cloning your bright spots. I want you to stop for a second to allow yourself to think. If you think with a clear head, you will make rational decisions rather than emotional ones. You enable the rider to control the elephant and steer it in the correct direction. The last thing you wish is to begin your weight loss journey heading down the wrong road. Your emotional thinking is six times stronger than your rational thinking, but this doesn't mean it's always right. In fact, it's nearly always wrong. This is why you need to stop to think; otherwise, the rider will never be able to control the sheer power of the elephant and lead it to your destination. Once the elephant settles, you will find that it will be more than happy to continue the journey as it will begin to see that it is moving closer towards the destination. Remember your growth mindset, where you believe you're good at some things. Your bright spots are those things. A part of a growth mindset is stopping to think about what you're doing well so you can congratulate yourself for what you're currently good at. Investigating these positive actions and experiences and cloning them creates more positive emotions and feelings. If you're sat here now and believe there is nothing you're good at, that's a fixed mindset. There are plenty of things you are currently good at which you can investigate and clone. You need to gain a growth mindset by finding even just one thing. Positive actions breed positive emotions, leading to truly remarkable results, and it all begins with following your bright spots.

Your To-Do List

1. Discover your bright spots. Find what you're currently doing well.

2. Study your bright spots. What makes these parts of your life easy and successful
3. Clone your bright spots. How can you replicate these positive actions?

7

FIND THE FEELING

PART ONE
SETTING YOUR GOALS

Saying you want to lose weight isn't enough; it is a present feeling. It doesn't stick with you throughout your weight loss journey or your lifetime. Further down the line, you won't feel like losing weight even though you want to. You give up and stop working towards your weight loss goal because saying you want to lose weight doesn't stick. There's no long-term feeling behind those words. It doesn't mean anything. In all my years working in the industry, when I ask anybody about their goal, they say, "I want to lose weight and tone up". I'm sure that's your goal too, but it doesn't mean anything. It's like saying, "I want to eat";

FIND THE FEELING

it's too vague. You need to be more specific and create goals that are unique to you. In this chapter, you will make "I want to lose weight and tone up" turn into a feeling within you that will help you lose and keep control of your weight for the rest of your life. You will never have to try to lose weight ever again.

In the health and fitness industry, they talk about SMART goals— Specific, Measurable, Attainable, Realistic, and Time. Saying I want to lose weight and tone up is none of these. This acronym is an excellent place to start when thinking about weight loss, as it allows you to create a stronger goal. You're encouraged to be more specific. What exactly do you wish to achieve? Go into as much detail as you possibly can. How much weight do you want to lose? Which areas of the body do you wish to tone up? What clothing size would you feel comfortable in? How would you like to feel?

You then decide how to measure your progress along the way. Are you going to weigh yourself weekly or daily? Are you going to take a monthly progress photo? How often are you going to record your measurements? Then, it would help to consider whether your goal is attainable. Is five stone in weight loss too much if you weigh thirteen stone? Then, you decide if your goal is realistic based on the lifestyle you wish to live. Can you attend the gym five times a week when you have a family at home and a career? Is clean eating every day realistic when you're a social butterfly? Finally, you then think about the time period of achieving your goal. Are you expecting to accomplish too much in too little time? Is two stone in two months a stretch? Is it sensible to aim for one stone lost in two months instead?

Although SMART goals are an excellent place to start as they get you thinking, your goal needs more than these rational questions and answers. This is why people still don't achieve their weight loss goal when they follow the SMART principle. Specific, Measurable, Attainable, Realistic, and Time framed doesn't mean anything within you. It makes sense when you think about it, and it appears to help, but it isn't exciting and doesn't get your emotions going. It's like how I'd imagine an accountancy Christmas party to be. The best way to achieve your weight loss goal with ease and simplicity is to motivate the elephant; to do this, you need to find the feeling. A feeling within you that's so strong it will stick with you every step of the way. Motivating the elephant so much that the rider can steer it in the correct direction without any resistance. You will begin by discovering exactly why you wish to lose weight, helping create a deeper meaning to your journey and a drive to succeed.

The next step is creating a step-by-step structure for your weight loss journey by setting behavioural goals that allow you to take action. You can change them in your current lifestyle to help you achieve your weight loss goal. Once you've created your action plan, it's time to set motivational goals that excite you every month, giving you something to work towards that isn't associated with what it says on the scales. If you only set a goal to lose weight, there is no structure to help you get there. Setting the goal types in this chapter allows you to measure your progress.

FIND THE FEELING

By the end of month one, you know whether you're on track and have a new motivational goal to boost you during month two. The more weight you have to lose, the more important it is to measure your progress, as it keeps you on track. Clear goals allow success to happen, ensuring you reach your weight loss goal.

Not having a strong enough goal happens all of the time, and it's so simple to change. If you don't find the feeling within you and set strong enough goals, you go into your weight loss journey half-hearted. There is no strong goal or deep motivating reason to get your head down and achieve it. Due to this, you aren't consistent with the actions needed to help you lose weight. Some days, you feel like it; others don't. You try one week, not the next, creating inconsistency and weight fluctuations. When you hit a problem on your journey, such as a week away or a night out, it sends you entirely off track. You don't notice your weight dropping as much as you'd like as it keeps going up and down in the same weight range, causing you to give up. You're tired of feeling like you're trying but not succeeding, and believe you will be this way for the rest of your life. This is not the case— You don't have a strong enough goal.

Before you set your goals, I want to say this to you. Whatever you do, don't follow the flock. I don't mean to sound insulting, but one thing that always happens is following the flock and setting goals similar to others. Yes, everybody who reads this book has the same goal of losing weight; however, finding the feeling is about finding the feeling within yourself. The only way to do this is to think about what it is you want to achieve and why you want to achieve it. If you say things because that's what you feel you should say and do things because other people are doing them, then it won't work. Your emotional, behavioural and motivational goals need to be unique to you. Instead of following the flock, I need you to be the best ewe can be.

Finding your why

I don't know whether you've ever encountered or heard of the five whys in other parts of your life, but they are how you will create your emotional goal. Everyone is always focused on what they want rather than why they want it. It's all well and good to say what you want to achieve, but a group cover of Billie Pipers 'Because We Want To' isn't going to cut it when answering the question 'Why Do You Want To Lose Weight?'. There are many flaws with only focusing on what you want to achieve and having a blasé response to why you want to lose weight. This is why you need to discover the deep meaning. Your wants may change over time; however, your why won't. Your wants won't hold you accountable and allow you to push through tricky times, but your why will. German philosopher Friedrich Nietzsche once said, "He who has a why to live can bear almost any how".

Your journey will be smooth, but this doesn't mean that you don't need to find your why and will get by with just a need to lose weight. Your journey becomes smooth because you will have a strong enough reason why you wish to lose weight. You won't have to bear almost any how due to your why, but you will be able to. Life is all about planning for the worst, to make anything less feel easy. Finding your why is part of your arsenal. Finding your why is one of the simplest things to do. All you need to do is ask yourself 'why' five times.

People don't need to know your true why. The main thing is that you discover your own why. Speaking about or being open about your true feelings can be scary, which is why many people feel uncomfortable discovering their own why. If you find the courage to be open to yourself and others, you will feel stronger and more confident that you can lose weight and keep it off. It helps if people close to you know the true reason you wish to lose weight, and this task is best done by having someone ask you 'why' so you react to the questions asked out loud. If you don't want to get somebody involved, write down the following question and answer it yourself. Here's an example of how it works.

First - Why do you want to lose weight?

Well, I feel sluggish and tired at my current weight.

Second - Why do you feel sluggish and tired at your current weight?

Simple tasks like walking up the stairs or playing with my kids are challenging.

Third - Why do you want to make these tasks easier?

Well, I want to make these tasks easier so I can do more.

Fourth - Why do you want to do more?

Well, I can't do as much each day, and I can't do as much with the kids these days.

Fifth - And why does that bother you?

Because I want to be an active parent and a role model for my kids. It's frustrating when they want to play sports in the garden, and I can't join in. I want to be a family that does fun activities together, and at the moment, I get out of breath. We can't do all of these things together.

There you have it. With just five questions, you've discovered the deep underlying factor as to why you want to lose weight. As you can see, it's more than just wanting to lose weight to look good or be healthy; it's this deep motivating factor that will be with you every step of the way. As I mentioned earlier, each person who reads this book will have the same goal of wanting to lose weight. However, the beauty of the five whys is that each person will have a different why unique to them.

Behavioural Goals

Behavioural goals are the actions needed to help you achieve your weight loss goal. They are black-and-white goals that don't allow any wiggle room. They are how you act. You do them, or you don't; it's that simple. I want you to think about your current behaviours. Are they helping or hindering your progress? A lot of the time, we want to achieve things, yet we aren't willing to change the behaviours that are needed to achieve them. There are many behavioural goals, and you must identify your current behaviours and decide how to set goals to create more positive behaviours. Let's look at some examples I've split into three categories— Mindset, Food and Exercise/Activity.

Mindset behavioural goals

"I will think positively and believe in myself."

If you set this goal and any negative thoughts occur in your journey, it's your job to tweak them and look at the positive.

"I will try everything at least once."

This goes for all types of exercise and even foods. Our taste buds alter over time, and our preferences for activities change too throughout our lifetime. Have an open mind and give everything a go at least once.

"I will get back on board immediately."

If you slip up by eating something you shouldn't have or skip an exercise session, don't worry about it. Just get back on board immediately and prevent it from going into the next meal or day.

"I will plan my week in advance."

You can be proactive rather than reactive. If you set this as a behavioural goal, you can proactively plan your meals and when you exercise that day.

Food behavioural goals

"I am going to cook all meals from scratch."

This states that you won't buy any packaged foods or meals on the go.

"I will reduce the number of sugary drinks."

You decide to reduce your sugary drinks week by week gradually.

"I will ensure I have plenty of vegetables with each meal."

You decide which vegetables you consume with each meal, putting these on your plate first.

Exercise and activity behavioural goals

"I will allocate three thirty-minute slots to exercise."

You put them in your diary and don't allow anything to take over them. You treat them like any other meeting or appointment. Once they are in the diary, you stick to them.

"I will take myself out of my comfort zone."

You ensure that each exercise session you do challenges you and takes you out of your comfort zone.

"I will do it even when I don't want to."

You ensure you do your planned exercise or activity, even when you don't feel like it or aren't motivated.

While reading through the above examples, I'm sure you have been thinking about how you can set behavioural goals related to you. They aren't exactly exciting, but they are essential. What behavioural goals can you set for yourself to hold you accountable and take action?

Motivational Goals

Motivational goals are the ones that are fun to work towards. They make you feel excited that you're about to achieve something that you've never been able to do before. Your weight loss journey will take some time, and by setting small targets to work towards each month, you can celebrate your wins more regularly rather than waiting until you achieve your final weight loss target. Motivational goals also create a sense of achievement. You feel so happy with yourself for achieving them, which becomes contagious. These small wins and feelings of positivity make weight loss easy and enjoyable. Each time you achieve something exciting, belief in yourself grows, strengthening the growth mindset. You're so set on getting that achievement high that you overcome barriers without even noticing they're potential barriers. Motivational goals allow you to focus on enjoying the journey rather than concentrating solely on the end result. Before you know it, you will have enjoyed the journey and arrive at your weight loss destination in no time.

Now you understand motivational goals, it's time to show you how to set them. The first question you must ask yourself is, 'What gets you excited?'. Take a moment to think about the question. Is it a feeling within yourself? A sense of achievement in your exercise sessions? A new adventure with your family, such as a bike ride or a holiday? It can be anything that gets you interested and excited to achieve that isn't associated with the number it says on the scales. Motivational goals are fun; without them, your journey would be monotonous and slow, so you need to stop and think about what motivates you. Here's an example of motivational goals for the first four months of an individual's journey.

Month One - I will be able to run for 10 minutes.

Month Two - I will be wearing a smaller clothing size.
Month Three - I will have more energy to be more active.
Month Four - I will be more confident in myself and my own ability.

I've outlined four types of motivational goals to give you an idea of the range within this type of goal setting. It's good to have different types at different markers. Each of us has our own factors that drive us to achieve things. It would help if you considered these motivational factors during your weight loss journey, as they are there to keep you going and remain motivated at all times. What motivational goals can you set to ensure you can celebrate small wins throughout your journey

Before you go and set your own goals, you must ensure you make them strong. A strong emotional goal will be with you during every step of your weight loss journey, and it's the sole reason why you will be driven to succeed. When you don't feel like exercising or are tempted by not-so-smart foods, remember your why. Your behavioural goals are needed as they will change you for the better. They aren't supposed to be thrillers, but they will encourage you to take action to move closer towards your weight loss goal. The final thing is to ensure your motivational goals get you excited and off your seat. A motivational goal excites you and gives you something to work towards that isn't associated with what it says on the scales. If it doesn't excite you, you need to adjust your goals. These three goals combined will create a feeling

FIND THE FEELING

within you that you can do this, but visualising your goals will really get you to find the feeling.

To find the feeling within you, imagine how it feels when you achieve your goals. When you've hit the milestones along the way, and once you've achieved your final weight loss goal. Visualising achieving your goals brings these feelings to life. Words on paper become feelings, and feelings become a reality. Do you remember when I said that achieving anything in life begins with the mind in the Grow Yourself chapter? Achieving your dreams starts with imagining the end result in your mind. Once you've set your goals, you must visualise achieving them.

You can begin this right now by visualising what it feels like to achieve your ultimate weight loss goal. What does it feel like? What do you look like? What compliments are people giving to you? How is your lifestyle now compared to how it was previously? Visualise achieving your goal in as much detail as possible. It's always important to visualise the milestones along the way. You can do that once you've created your motivational and behavioural goals. Your journey could take months or even over a year, so it is important to visualise achieving each of your motivational goals to create a feeling of excitement within you.

The number it says on the scales is just a number. Yes, you wish to lose a particular number of stones or pounds, but it doesn't spark a feeling within you as it's just a statement. This is why I encourage people to take progress photos each month to see how their weight loss has altered their body shape. Having something that shows you how far you've come is also a good idea. I know we appear to live in a cashless society these days, but I always recommend using pound coins to represent each pound of body weight you wish to lose. Let's say you're looking to lose two stone, which is twenty-eight pound. Place twenty-eight-pound coins in a jar on a windowsill, fireplace or worktop. At the same time, have another empty jar at the end of where you display your jars. Every time you lose one pound, move one pound coin from the jar with twenty-eight pounds to the empty jar. If you lose two pounds in one week, shift two-pound coins over. Equally, if you gain one pound, then you shift a pound back to the original jar. Your goal is to switch all twenty-eight-pound coins to the other jar. This may sound a little silly, but it allows you to see how far you've come and allows you to see how many pounds you've lost physically. This will hold you accountable if you gain weight and motivate you when you lose weight. You will find a feeling within you when you see the pounds moving from one jar to the other.

    The pound coins in a jar is a great way to visualise your progress, and you must visualise achieving your goal in a physical way too. Is there a particular item of clothing you can't wait to wear once you reach your weight loss goal? If you own it, I want you to get it out of the wardrobe. If you don't own it, it sounds like an excuse for some retail therapy. Could you go and buy it now? Don't get ahead of yourself and go on a shopping spree; you only need one item. Once you have the item, I want you to hang it up. Not in your wardrobe, but in a place where you can see it every day so each time you walk past it, you find the feeling within you to keep working towards your goal. Just like the pound coins, it may seem silly to get an item of clothing out of the wardrobe when you aren't going to be wearing it for a while, but it works wonders.

Visualising aims to bring your dreams into reality, and physical props are perfect to spark these positive emotions within you. It also doesn't have to be a piece of clothing. A photo of your holiday destination pinned on the fridge will help you find the feeling each time you see it. You can use the clothing prop upstairs and the holiday destination in the kitchen. A couple of props in different places around the house work too. What physical item will you use to visualise achieving your weight loss goal?

Your To-Do List

1. Find your why. The deep motivating reason as to why you want to lose weight.
2. Set your behavioural goals. The positive actions that will help you move closer to your weight loss goal.
3. Set your motivational goals. The exciting and mini goals that help you stay motivated throughout your journey.

PART TWO
FIND SOMETHING YOU LOVE

In the Grow Yourself chapter, I encouraged you to be more active. I provided you with key examples of exercise styles you could do. When reading about interval training, lifting weights or walks in the park, did you get super excited to do them? I'm assuming not. We are often led to believe the best and only way to exercise is by joining a gym. But do you even like going? I've worked in gyms over the years, and I can't say they feel like the most welcoming or motivating environments to be in. I'm guessing you're not a fan either? It's rare to find the feeling within you when staring at a wall while running on the treadmill for thirty minutes.

People always view exercise and its efforts as a chore. As something you've got to do. If you've read the previous paragraph and thought there's nothing you will love, then don't worry. Part two of Find The Feeling aims to help you

FIND THE FEELING

find something you love, and to do this, you need to be open-minded. There's something out there for everyone. Part of developing a growth mindset is being open-minded. A person with a fixed mindset will say they don't like something before they've even tried it, but you can only come to that conclusion once you've given it a go. Someone with a growth mindset will get themselves out there, be open-minded and try it before they have an opinion. If you didn't like something in the past but you've not done it for a long time, I'd encourage you to go out there and try it again. You never know, you may like it this time. Believing the gym is the only option for exercising is being narrow-minded. There are so many other ways of exercising, and there are so many different ways of being more active too. You must get out there and try as many of them as possible. Enjoy trying new things, and you never know; you may find something you love.

To exercise regularly, you must find something you love doing. Something that makes you happy and provides a positive feeling when participating in that activity. If you find something you love, you will look forward to doing it and can't wait to participate in the activity you've chosen. If you enjoy it and can't wait to participate, you will consistently do this form of exercise. You will also miss it when you're unable to do it. This is always a good sign you've found something you love when you get annoyed for being unable to do it. As you love doing it, it's more than exercise. It becomes a hobby, an interest, or a social event. It becomes who you are as a person instead of the chore you once believed exercise had to be. It reduces stress, increases happiness, and provides a strong social aspect to your life. When you're happy and less stressed, the results will come flying in.

If you don't find something you love, you may do what most people do and join the local gym, where they believe they must go to exercise. In pillar three of the Grow Yourself chapter, I mentioned three ways of exercising that all sounded like they needed to be done in a gym when they can be done in various places. Let's say you decide to join a gym. You may go religiously for a week or two, but the novelty soon disappears. The honeymoon period ends, and you find you weren't enjoying it. It's busy and full of posers taking selfies. The equipment is sweaty, and you are confused about what to do there. All of this puts you off, even though you joined with the best intentions, and you stop going. Instead of the positive emotions and excellent results you thought you would have, you feel defeated and uncomfortable, and to make matters even worse, you're tied to a twelve-month membership.

Don't worry, though. It's not your fault, and you're not alone. You did what everybody else does. I used to look after five hundred members in an exclusive gym, and only around eighty people had visited the gym in the last three months. That's unbelievable when gym membership costs a lot of money, but it happens at every single gym around the world. They make more money from people who don't even attend, which is why you tend to be signed up on a twelve-month contract. If you want to go to the gym, you can go, but it doesn't have to be the gym if you don't want it to be. If you're unsure what you could love, let's look at what you could do. I've split exercise and activity into three sections — Sports, Activities, and Home Workouts.

Are there sports you love?

I bet you never thought you would read about sports in this book, but it's always a good place to begin when searching for something you love. Do you enjoy watching the Tennis at Wimbledon every Summer? When you watch it, have you ever said, "We should go and play tennis at the park"? If so, go and give it a try with a friend or family member. Are your kids football-mad? If they're always asking you to take them to the park, can you have a kick around with them and enjoy some family time? Did you used to play a sport for the team at school? Can you browse the internet to see if a local team needs a new player? These examples show you that there are many options to be more active and find something you love within sports. It all begins with listening for opportunities and thinking about what you enjoy.

A sport is a game. When playing, you focus on the game instead of the exercise you're doing. It covers the fact that you're exercising and pushes you to try harder than a typical exercise session, as you will be focused on winning the next point, beating your opponent, or scoring a goal. They provide you with a feeling of achievement if you win and the motivation to do better and improve if you lose. The social factor plays a key role in why many people participate in sports. Sports provide a sociable way to exercise, such as competing on a team or individually against an opponent. You interact with team members when playing and build relationships, becoming friends outside of the sport. They are fun to participate in, and the beauty of sports is that there is something out there for everyone, regardless of age or ability. There are so many sports for you to try, participate in, and fall in love with.

Team sports - Netball, Football, Rugby, Hockey, Volleyball, Lacrosse, Basketball, Cricket
Individual sports - Tennis, Badminton, Squash, Archery and Table Tennis, Golf, Running, Swimming, Yoga, Climbing, Surfing,
Group sports - Gymnastics, Dancing, Cycling, Boxing, CrossFit, Judo, Kickboxing, Weightlifting, Horse Riding and Athletics

I didn't want to bombard you with endless examples; you get the gist. If you're thinking of something I have yet to mention, go and give it a go if you will love it.

Are there activities you love?

If sports are a big no-no, why don't you try and give a variety of activities a go? It goes without saying that we don't get outside enough these days. The true beauty of our parks, countryside, rivers and canals supply us with multiple areas to exercise when we get outside and away from the roads. Something is calming about being outdoors and away from everything. It helps you enjoy the activity more and affects your stress levels. Outdoor activities such as a countryside walk, mountain biking, kayaking, open water swimming or paddleboarding are great places to start. My dog would disagree with the paddleboarding suggestion, but each to their own. If you have kids, get involved in family activities like going to the park, camping, bowling, mini golf or trampolining.

If you like gardening, make it a part of your routine, or if you're good with a toolbox, do some DIY. If you're house proud, get involved in cleaning more regularly. There's something therapeutic about hoovering the floor and scrubbing kitchen works tops. If you're into cars, make washing the car part of your weekly routine. These activities that you already do are bright spots, which are always a great place to start being more active. Indoor activities include dancing to your favourite music, exercising with the kids, meditating to decrease stress levels, and practising your putting in the hallway. You'd be surprised how many extra steps you take walking up and down the hall. You could also do regular stretching sessions to feel stiffness and pain-free. The suggestions could go on. If you think there's something else you could love doing, go and give it a try.

Are there home workouts you love?

The other and more traditional option is home workouts. These are the closest to exercise sessions in a gym but in the comfort and privacy of your own home. The rise of technology such as YouTube and smart TVs allows you to enjoy the feeling of a class environment without leaving

FIND THE FEELING

your house. Some people love working out but feel uncomfortable doing it in front of others. I love singing, but I'm not willing to belt out Lewis Capaldi songs if there are other people around. Others love dancing, but if their favourite song comes on at a wedding, they may be uncomfortable getting up and letting loose unless they've had a few too many G&Ts. Doing a dance workout at home allows you to dance like nobody is watching, because they aren't.

Home workouts are also such a practical way of being more active. You turn on the TV, and you're off. We all live busy lives, which can be a problem when allocating time to exercise. There's no travel time or childcare issues, eliminating a potential barrier for many people. People love this freedom to mix up their workouts and be free and comfortable at home. You can try a yoga class and do a downward dog with the dog. Do a dance class with the kids or stick a HIIT workout on if you're short of time. Finding something you love is about finding something that works for you.

Finding the feeling is about more than just being active. It's about improving your mental health by getting outdoors and clearing your mind. It's about doing something for yourself. It's socialising with friends, family and like-minded people. Relationships strengthen as your health improves. If you do what you love, you will enjoy it more, meaning you will do it more. It's always good to do something you love as you will make time to do it and be more consistent. Mix it up and try new things to keep life fresh and exciting. Refrain from going into your new way of exercising and think of it as just exercise. Be open-minded, smile, enjoy yourself, get involved and work hard. All these things mean you will stick to a routine because it's much more than just burning calories. Whatever you do, don't hold back and never doubt your ability. Find something you love.

Your To-Do List

1. Ask yourself, What do you love? Take a moment to think about what you love or used to love doing.
2. Ask yourself, What could I try? Approach it with an open mind and think about some new things you could try.
3. Think about what you're going to do. Decide what you will do as some form of activity or exercise.

8

SHRINK THE CHANGE

When you analyse a problem, do you seek a solution that befits the scale of it? I'm asking you this question because it's such a common issue that needs to be addressed. We look at a big goal, such as losing weight, and feel we must fix it with a big, outlandish solution. You see the amount of weight you wish to lose and feel you must turn your life upside down. You begin exercising every day, say no to all of the foods you enjoy and say yes to kale smoothies. You try to live the life of an Olympic athlete overnight. Although I don't think even they have kale smoothies. More weight to lose doesn't mean the solution needs to be bigger. You must understand that everybody's weight loss journey should be treated the same. If you have more to lose, it will just take a little longer.

We always rush to lose weight and want results as quickly as possible. Unrealistic expectations and nonsensical instructions have plagued Weight Loss. Everybody believes that they must rush off and try and do as much as they can as quickly as possible. Still, consider how long it took to gain weight and be patient when working towards your weight loss goal. It's going to take time. If you've been skipping the tasks at the end of each chapter, slow down and do things step by step. There's no point in reading this book if you don't take action at the end of each chapter.

One thing that ceases to amaze me is the lengths people go to overcomplicate the simplest tasks. The weight loss process is one of them. As you're working through these chapters, you're beginning to realise that weight loss is a pretty simple process, and nothing is impressive about complicating it. You track your calories to ensure you're in a calorie deficit, provide your body with nutrient-rich foods, believe you can lose weight, and aim to be more active. If it's so simple, why do people start a weight loss journey and try and overcomplicate things? It may be intentional as they feel there is something impressive when they tell their friends how they're following Keto. It may be an unintentional way for them to feel like they need to be punished, so they are super strict with what they can eat and when. They think doing more will deliver more, yet it's quite the opposite.

The more complicated a task is, the more likely a person will fail. If you've failed at losing weight in the past, you must use your growth mindset to learn from these previous failures. Were you trying to do too much? Did it not fit into your lifestyle? Was the timing not right? Why do you think you've failed? You can learn so much from your previous failures, and one of them you should remember

SHRINK THE CHANGE

is that doing too much backfires. Life is simple, but humans overcomplicate things. The Rider in you knows that complicated doesn't work, yet the Elephant feels you should be doing more. The Rider gets overruled each time you try to lose weight, even though your emotions don't like big obstacles, and the logical decision is to make things easier for yourself. The only way to make change easier is to learn how to be a good rider and motivate the Elephant. To do this, you must shrink the change.

Have you ever seen an elephant win the hurdles? If the elephant were to ever compete in such an event, it would be near impossible to get over the first hurdle. If it somehow managed to leap like Colin Jackson over the first, it would be so fatigued from such a surprising leap that it would struggle to repeat it for a further nine hurdles. This is what happens when you try to make big changes over and over again. You may do it once, but you won't be able to keep it up, meaning you won't make it to the finish line. The only way for the Elephant to complete the event is to lower the hurdles so much that it can easily step over them. Although the elephant feels it should make difficult changes, it also likes changes it can make. The Rider must direct the Elephant over the low hurdles rather than the high ones. It might feel like it should try to be an athlete and go over the big ones. Still, once it realises that it has gone past a barrier that it previously had to stop at, it will become more motivated and more content with following this new road.

Insanity is doing the same thing over and over again and expecting different results. You've broken the chain and are working your way through a different approach, so you can now expect different results than that of your previous failed attempts. While others are rushing around, making things really difficult for themselves, you can follow your own route, knowing it will work. You understand that achieving your weight loss goal can be simple. Simplicity is the ultimate sophistication, which lies in shrinking the change. Each time you change something, ask yourself, "Is this change so small and easy that an elephant could step over it?" Are these changes so small that your emotions are unfazed by them?

Weight loss is more achievable when making just one change at a time. It allows you to focus all your energy and attention on one thing, making it more manageable. Tiny changes collectively create big results. Your big weight loss goal is slowly chipped away without spooking the elephant. Preventing it from running off in the wrong direction. Small changes allow you to remain calm and positive because you know you're heading in the right direction and are getting closer to your weight loss goal. Earlier, you set motivational and behavioural goals that allow you to celebrate lots of mini-wins along the way. Smaller changes are potential behavioural goals you can add to your list. It's always better to celebrate lots of mini-wins throughout your weight loss journey rather than waiting for the big win of achieving your ultimate weight loss goal. We all lead busy lives, and trying to drastically change everything in your life is impractical. Shrinking the change allows you to achieve your weight loss goal practically. One that fits into your current lifestyle rather than forcing you to live a lifestyle you don't wish to live.

If you're still considering making drastic changes, think of how it will go. You may get somewhere, but you won't achieve your ultimate goal. You will start by trying to change everything at once. You make all the changes you can make and drastically change your lifestyle, believing that's what will get you the results you've always dreamed of. You soon realise that it isn't a sustainable way and find it hard to stick to the changes that you're trying to make. You're frustrated, lose motivation, and the Elephant within you is spooked and runs off due to your emotions getting the better of you. Any progress you've made is lost, and you end up back where you started. You wait until you're recharged and motivated to try again before you repeat the same mistakes. You remain stuck in this cycle and never make it to your weight loss goal.

Now that you know the importance of shrinking the change and making just one change at a time, it's time to think about what needs to change. I encourage you not to get overwhelmed with all the things you could change. Remember, everything doesn't and shouldn't be changed at once. It would help if you looked at all aspects of your life. Which parts of your lifestyle need to change to help you lose weight? Is it your food, an increase in activity or exercise, or a change in your work or social life? Look at what needs to change in each area, as this will allow you to shrink the change so it feels more achievable and doesn't spook the elephant. There are so many things you could change, but you need to think about what needs to change to allow you to move forward and closer towards your weight loss goal. What you could change and need to change are entirely different things. Let's take a look at some examples of each area.

There are many things you could change concerning food. Some are eating behaviours like eating slowly and mindfully, putting your knife and fork down until you've chewed and swallowed your previous mouthful, and eating at the table without distractions. These eating-habit behavioural changes make a massive difference in how much you eat. Don't believe me? Go and give it a try. Small changes create big results. Cooking and preparation-related behaviours include cooking all meals yourself so you know what's in each meal. A beneficial change could be to measure food quantities to reduce your overall portion sizes. Many people eat the correct things, but their portions are too large. Measuring things like rice, pasta, and oats allows you to see a true serving size. Then there are types of foods you could change. Consuming smart food choices over not-so-smart food choices are small changes that shrink the change.

Activity-related changes are things that seem too simple or minor to help you lose weight; however, when done daily, they compound and make weight loss easier to achieve. These include walking instead of driving to close places, taking the stairs instead of the lift, playing with your kids at the park instead of watching them and spending more time standing than sitting. Another one that may not be related directly to activity is getting sufficient sleep because when you are more energised, you will be more willing to move. Sleeping more will also mean you won't crave as many sugary foods too, so add an extra thirty minutes to your sleep time and see how much it returns.

Exercise-related changes are things like exercising for ten minutes a day to keep you feeling productive and healthy. A change could be to include resistance exercises in your workouts to help tone and build more muscle to look great, feel strong and increase your metabolism. If you're already exercising, a small change that will make a big difference is ensuring you're exercising at a challenging intensity. If you do this, you will burn more calories in the same duration. Taking a look at your diary and allocating time to exercise each week to be more consistent with your workouts is also an organisational change you could make with regard to exercise.

Changes you could make in your work and social life will also help you lose weight. Social-related changes could be reducing the number of times you eat out in restaurants, reducing your weekly alcohol intake or socialising over activities rather than food or drink. Creating a positive and strong support structure around you and saying no to things that don't help you on your weight loss journey is a social change with plenty of rewards.

Work-related changes include ensuring you do a ten-minute workout before checking your emails in the morning, making your lunch to take into work with you, or setting a behavioural goal, such as prioritising an evening run over extra work you've taken home and aren't getting paid extra for. As you can see, there are many small changes you can make in various parts of your life that will help you shrink the change and move further down the road to weight loss.

Once you've thought about what needs to change, the next question is —What are you willing to trade? As change is all about trade-offs. Our lives are made up of lots of different actions. As individuals, we choose what actions to partake in, with some being good and others bad. Some help, and others hinder progress. Saying yes to one thing means saying no to another. When you change something, you say no to something old and yes to something new. These trade-offs can cause issues because we don't want to give up certain things. This can be scary to the Elephant as it likes to feel comfortable and stick with what they already do and know. For change to happen, both the Elephant and the Rider must be willing to make them. This is why it's crucial to consider trade-offs you may or may not be willing to make throughout your weight loss journey. Let's take a look at some examples of trade-offs.

- Saying yes to getting more sleep means saying no to watching another episode on Netflix.
- Saying yes to going for a run means saying no to thirty minutes of browsing the Internet.
- Saying yes to preparing your meals at home means saying no to picking up food on the go because it's practical.

- Saying yes to a slower and more sustainable approach means saying no to crash diets and ridiculous training plans.
- Saying yes to reducing your alcohol intake means saying no to meeting your friend in the pub for a mid-week drink.
- Saying yes to your way of doing things means saying no to listening to what those around you are doing.
- Saying yes to losing weight means saying no to the treats brought into the office.

There are so many trade-offs you could decide to make, and these examples clearly show that saying yes to one thing means saying no to another. When you agree to a new change, think about what you are saying no to and decide whether you can and are willing to say no. Small changes lead to small victories, often triggering improved behaviour and compliance. If you make just one small change you're willing to make, you will see excellent results without much effort. It's efficiency at its finest. I know I've said it many times throughout this chapter, but I'll repeat it—Only focus on one change at a time. Focusing on more than one change can be tempting, but think of it like juggling balls. One is easy, and two is manageable with effort. Three balls, you may drop them all and have to start again, and any more is just ridiculous. Juggle one ball at a time, make one change at a time, and make things easier for yourself.

SHRINK THE CHANGE

Many of us think that we are above simple and take pride in the fact that we make things complicated. We love to tell people how hard something is and try to impress them with fancy weight loss methods and complex jargon. Complexity creates complications, and we don't want that. Think of the bigger picture. Think eight weeks, six months, or even a year down the line. Imagine how much further along the road to weight loss you would be with steady, incremental changes done consistently. Shrink the change and make sure you master each change before moving on to the next one. It may not seem like it's doing much at first, but it will compound over time if you stick to it and it allows you to make it to your destination.

Your To-Do List

1. List all of the changes that you could make. What changes could you make to help you lose weight?
2. Think about what you're willing to trade. What are you willing to say yes to, and what are you willing to say no to?
3. Think about what needs to change. Are there any changes that are essential in ensuring you lose weight?

9

SCRIPT THE CRITICAL MOVES

Shrinking the change allows you to think of plenty of tiny changes that compound together over time to create remarkable results. After completing the task, you will have a long list of all of the changes you could make. You've also created a large inventory of all the things you could possibly trade, but the problem with large lists is that they can cause you to feel overwhelmed. You either procrastinate because you don't know which to make off your extensive list, or you panic and begin making a few changes at a time. Neither of these situations help you. This is why it's important not only to shrink the changes you make but to script the critical moves that will propel you in the direction of your weight loss goal. Scripting the critical moves is where you'll filter the potential changes

SCRIPT THE CRITICAL MOVES

you could make into the critical ones that will help you the most.

In the previous chapter, you understood that saying yes to one thing means saying no to the other, and you discovered what needs to change. When making any change in your life, you must ask yourself the following three questions. To make change easy, you must be able to say you're a nine or ten out of ten in response to each question. Easy changes mean an easy weight loss journey, and it all begins with being willing, able, and ready to change.

How willing are you to make this change?

The key question when aiming to make change easy is how willing you are to make it. For easy change to happen, you must be willing to make it. If you aren't willing, it will be difficult to make it successfully, so what's the point of trying? Think back to saying yes to one thing means saying no to another in the previous chapter. There are some things you aren't willing to change yet. Only focus on the things that you are willing to change. Ask yourself how willing you are to make the change on a scale of 1 to 10 and only make the change if the answer is a nine or ten. If the answer isn't a nine or ten, move on to another change you are willing to make. If you find yourself unwilling to make any changes, this isn't going to work. It would be best to go back to discovering your why and ensure it's the deep motivating factor that inspires change. It would also be best to go back and think about how you can gain a growth mindset too. I've had clients say no to everything when asked if they're willing to change, and I've also had clients say yes to everything when asked the same question but have not meant their answer. Only make a change if you're honestly willing to make it. If the answer is a nine or ten, move on to the next question.

How able are you to make this change?

Unfortunately, our circumstances don't allow us to make the changes we are willing to make. This causes a barrier which you don't wish to have. We all have parts of our lives that we can't change at this moment in time. You don't need to worry about it right now. Instead, you can focus on it later if it matters at all. Your life might be so hectic with work or family commitments that you aren't able to get out and go for a run. If this is the case, you must aim to shrink the change and lower the barrier. If you can't get outside and are short on time, can you exercise indoors for ten minutes with your kids? If this allows you to answer the question with a nine or ten, meaning you're able to make the change, then make it. If you're still unable to make the change, don't make it. Only make the change if you're willing and able to make it. If the answer is a nine or ten, move on to the next question.

How ready are you to make this change?

When making any change, no matter how big or small, you must ask yourself if you're ready to make the change.

SCRIPT THE CRITICAL MOVES

Doing this will encourage you to hold yourself accountable and remain focused to make it. It will also prevent you from making the excuse that you aren't ready to make it as you've already decided you are before taking action. You should only make a change if you're ready to make it. On a scale of 1 to 10, ask yourself how ready are you to make the change. If the answer isn't a nine or ten, don't make that change.

This is how to keep things easy. If you ask yourself how willing you are, how able, and how ready you are to make a change, and the answer isn't a nine or a ten for each, don't make that particular change. Even if you feel you have to make it, you can only make it if you are willing, able, and ready to, as this is how to make change easy. There's no point in battling something that won't happen right now. You will tire yourself out, and there are obstacles along the way, causing weight loss to feel hard to achieve and even impossible. You must always follow the road of least resistance by focusing on the things you are ready to change, are willing to change and are able to change.

When you go for an eye test, you are asked to read the numbers from top to bottom. You begin with the biggest ones, the ones that are the easiest to read. You say a few big letters, and you're already halfway down the page without any effort to read them. When setting off on your weight loss journey, you must begin with the big moves that will help you move closer to your goal without any significant effort to make them. These fundamental

SCRIPT THE CRITICAL MOVES

changes propel you halfway down the road to achieving your weight loss goal. Unfortunately, we try to make the changes from the bottom of the page that don't move you closer to your goal. The changes from the bottom of the page are difficult to make and don't significantly affect your results. All that you gain from making them is short-term kudos from others. It's a weird world we live in when you get praised for making difficult and idiotic changes that don't help but don't get any recognition for making sensible and practical changes.

It would be best if you didn't strive for recognition from others for making silly and difficult changes. Your goal isn't to get all your friends to say how strong, committed, and resilient you are to make such difficult changes they couldn't make. This shouldn't be an ego-driven journey for recognition. It should be a purpose-driven journey for weight loss. If you do this, friends and family will recognise your achievements and praise you for doing well. Sticking at something is challenging for many people, and the results you've gained are what others want. Nobody wishes they could make difficult changes that don't mean anything. They just feel as though they should, but in the words of Beverley Knight, "Shoulda Woulda Coulda can't change your mind, And I wonder, wonder, wonder what I'm gonna do, Shoulda Woulda Coulda are the last words of a fool".

When you have a long list of all the possible changes you could make, you can easily be tempted not to think for yourself and go for the changes that everybody else is making. Remember, most people overlook the simplicity

SCRIPT THE CRITICAL MOVES

of weight loss and make overcomplicated and difficult changes. These changes only help a little and require many sacrifices, meaning your weight loss journey will be a hard slog. Your objective is to make weight loss easy by making simple changes that help a lot and don't require any significant sacrifices.

Let's say you make a change that isn't important for weight loss, such as eating so-called superfoods you don't like. You begin munching on kale and goji berries and hate every minute of it. You do it because you believe it's a change that will help, as everyone is always calling them superfoods that help with weight loss. You're trying hard to stick to this change, but due to no progress being made, you then make another change that doesn't matter and begin drinking apple cider vinegar. Unfortunately, this doesn't work even though you're trying even harder to lose weight. You make a third change and start doing some daily bicep curls and sit-ups to get the weight off. The exercises burn a few extra calories, and the kale and goji berries will provide some nutrients. Still, you've made three changes that don't deliver the expected results.

You've sacrificed so much but got nothing in return, which causes you to give up as you're tired and frustrated. Nobody can disregard your effort, but your execution was poor. Your energy and commitment have been channelled on things that don't matter. Instead, focusing on the most straightforward changes would be best. These are also the most efficient changes, giving you the biggest bang for your buck. Each bit of effort you put in will return twice the results you were expecting. They are the changes that matter and will significantly impact your weight loss journey.

I've structured this book to encourage you to focus on the most critical parts first. The critical move I started this book with was to track your calories and to ensure you track them consistently. This is the number one critical move for weight loss and maintenance. Focus on being consistent with this critical move, and then, once you are, add another critical move. If you need clarification on what changes are critical moves and which ones aren't, I have some examples.

Critical Move Examples

Tracking your calories consistently via MyFitnessPal — This is the most important critical move when starting your weight loss journey, which is why I started this book with a chapter all about it. It shows you the number of calories you're consuming compared to your calorie intake goal. Once you see the numbers, you can see if you will lose weight, gain, or stay the same. If you went over your calories one day, you can adjust the next day's intake to ensure you get back on track. Clicking and logging your food intake on your phone requires minimal effort and helps you lose weight enormously.

Preparing your own meals — We look at food as the same whether it's bought out and about or made at home, but have you ever bought a sandwich from a shop only to find it's got minimal filling but a ridiculous amount of calories in it compared to if you made it at home. Preparing your meals at home allows you to see how many calories and nutrients you put into your meal. It also allows you to have a more satisfying meal as you can put more filling in it and still consume fewer calories than if you bought your food out.

Eating slowly and mindfully — You will read this one and feel as though it doesn't sound like a critical move, but that's the thing about them; they don't seem much as they are easy to make. Eating slowly and mindfully are habits that allow you to identify what you're eating and allow your body time to decide when it is full. We will get to this later in the book, but we are so busy and distracted these days that our eating habits encourage us to consume more food than we need.

Increasing your activity levels — We've already mentioned increasing your activity levels to allow you to use more energy and feel better mentally and physically. If you don't exercise at all, doing just one thirty-minute exercise session per week is a critical move. You can alternatively do three ten-minute workouts per week. The critical move is increasing what you're doing. For some who are already regular exercisers, they could increase the intensity of their exercise sessions. For others, it might be a daily walk after dinner.

Not Critical Move Examples

Consuming so-called superfoods — I love kale, quinoa, and goji berries, but a superfood is just a marketing tool to promote a product or sell a magazine. All smart food choices are beneficial. Instead of consuming one of these superfoods, aim to move your food intake from the not-so-smart food choices to the smart food choices. That is a critical move.

Deciding whether to have a high-fat, low-carb diet or a low-fat, high-carb diet — The debate on whether a high-fat, low-carb diet or a low-fat, high-carb diet is better will continue forever. This is why it's not a critical move. Fats and carbohydrates provide the body with essential nutrients, so I recommend you consume them both. In my eyes, the debate is just a preference, so if you prefer more carbohydrates over fats or more fats over carbohydrates, it doesn't matter. What matters is that whatever food you eat keeps you under the calorie goal you set for yourself each day.

Deciding to drink apple cider vinegar or green tea — Whoever created this sorcery must be banned from associating these foods with weight loss. Any food that is isolated and branded as helping with weight loss should be prohibited. The body doesn't decide to lose weight because you've included one specific food. This is why it's not a critical move. If you like a cup of green tea, have one, but don't have one because you believe it will help you lose weight. What will help you lose weight is ensuring you're in a calorie deficit.

SCRIPT THE CRITICAL MOVES

Deciding to do a dumbbell chest press instead of using a barbell — This is just a move. It does not matter whatsoever. I've included this example because I get asked, "What are the best exercises to lose weight?" and "Will doing daily sit-ups help me burn belly fat?". The best exercises to lose weight are the ones you're most likely to stick to. For one person, it could be walking or water aerobics, and for the other, it could be spin classes and playing football. The priority with exercises is that you remain consistent with them to keep your activity levels up. Daily sit-ups won't help you lose belly fat. Sit-ups strengthen the muscles in your stomach, but they don't play a major part in burning the belly fat on top of it. What's critical to losing body fat is being in a calorie deficit. A critical move to help you lose belly fat would be to include some form of resistance training, such as squats, press-ups, lunges, and single-arm rows.

Critical moves are like taking an aeroplane to a different country. The not-so-important moves are like working out how to get from your room to the restaurant once you get to your destination. What this means is that the first moves you make are the ones that are going to get you quickly towards your destination as efficiently as possible. It's critical moves that will help you do this. When you look at all of the changes you could make, you must structure them in order of most effective and critical. Once you do this, you will soon see that most of the changes you could make don't matter at all, and you probably will never have to focus on making. Begin with the most critical move and

SCRIPT THE CRITICAL MOVES

ensure you can be at least 90% consistent with it. It may only take you one week to be consistent with it, or it may take you one month. Whatever you do, ensure you are 90% consistent with it. Only then can you move on to your second critical move. There are no time restrictions; this is all about consistency. It's not a competition on how many you've made compared to others, so don't be distracted by the number and type of changes others make. Focus on your critical moves and make the moves that will help you the most.

Now that you've shrunk the changes and have structured your critical moves, you should see how making the required changes is pretty straightforward. I need to finish this chapter by saying don't be attracted by shiny things. Shiny things can be anything. They can be a trend, a fad or something someone has told you. Shiny things are distractions, gossip, and myths. Things that make you go, "Oh, what's that? Should I be doing that now?". Just because someone is making a change that you're not, it doesn't mean you need to go out and make that change too. Just because you've heard that turmeric is good for weight loss, it doesn't mean that you need to start drinking turmeric lattes instead of your cup of Yorkshire tea. Just because someone you know has begun to wear a waist trainer doesn't mean you need to go out and buy one.

Focus on your changes and ask me in the forum on my website if you need clarification on whether the change you want to make is critical. It can feel like a move isn't critical because it doesn't feel challenging, but it will make the biggest difference. You've now decided which

SCRIPT THE CRITICAL MOVES

changes you will make and have discovered which ones are your critical moves. This is where you should be focusing your attention. Don't be attracted by shiny things. Refrain from being tempted by what other people are doing or saying. Remember, this is your weight loss journey, and you're doing what you believe is best for you.

Your To-Do List

1. Find your critical moves from the list of changes you could make after the shrink the change chapter.
2. Put them in order of most significant impact. Think smarter, not harder. It's all about efficiency. Which ones are going to help you progress the most?
3. Ask yourself how consistent you can be with each critical move. Can you be 90% consistent with each one?

10

POINT TO THE DESTINATION

PART ONE
PLANNING AHEAD

For some reason, we set off on our weight loss journey without knowing how to reach our destination. You wouldn't get in a car at Land's End with the destination being John O'Groats, and guess how to get there without using motorways. You'd use the sat nav to make your journey easy. It would set a clear route, show you the best way, and divert you around any obstacles, such as heavy traffic or road closures. This is what you need to do on your weight loss journey. It would be best to decide how you

POINT TO THE DESTINATION

would get to your destination by planning ahead and anticipating any obstacles along the way, allowing a smooth weight loss journey. The last thing you want is a stressful and bumpy ride full of obstacles and discomfort. Remember, keep asking yourself - What would your journey look like if it was easy? By continually asking yourself this question, you follow the road of least resistance. When there's no resistance, you will arrive at your destination before you know it.

Pointing to the destination is a chapter that teaches you how to be a good rider of the elephant, as you'll have mapped out a route that makes sense to follow. It also allows you to control the elephant and ensure you continue heading in the right direction. Planning your journey is the first part of the chapter that will help the rider within you point to the destination, allowing you to anticipate what will happen throughout your weight loss journey. By the time any roadblocks pop up, you've already anticipated them, so they don't phase you. Instead, you've already created a plan for this moment to help you continue moving forward with ease and without any negative feelings.

Suppose you're going out at the weekend and know that sticking to your calorie target may be tricky. In that case, you can reduce your daily calorie intake during the week ahead to balance the books. If you know that you have a busy period coming up, you can batch-cook healthy meals to put in the freezer, so all you have to do is microwave a meal, and you're still on track. These are just a couple of examples of planning your journey, anticipating potential issues, and creating a plan so they aren't a problem and you remain on track. When you do this, you stay in a mental state of focus and stillness. Instead of flapping, panicking and allowing other negative emotions to kick in, you realise you can remain on the correct road towards your weight loss destination. You already know everything that's about to happen during your journey.

You may be scared or overwhelmed at the thought of planning your weight loss journey and looking at everything that could get in your way. The belief that various barriers may prevent you from achieving your weight loss goal could make you think it's not worth trying. That is a fixed mindset; this thought will become your reality if you don't plan your journey. No matter how hard you try, things keep popping up out of nowhere, causing your weeks to become so unpredictable. Other parts of your life take over, steering you in the wrong direction and causing you to become frustrated with yourself. Your weight loss journey feels difficult and, at times, impossible to achieve. If you're ever left to choose between failure and success, which would you pick? It's your call. Failure is inevitable if you don't plan your weight loss journey and have a fixed mindset. Success is guaranteed if you map out your weight loss journey and have a growth mindset.

"If I had six hours to chop down a tree, I'd spend the first four hours sharpening the axe." This means that before you start working on a big task or challenge, you must take time to plan how you will do it. Although you won't take physical action as quickly as others, taking time to think about your approach pays off in the long run. When you take the sharpened axe and make the first

POINT TO THE DESTINATION

swing, it will slice through the tree like a knife through butter. You can't just go into things mindlessly and hope for the best. The people who set off before you will still be chipping away at bark even though they set off four hours earlier than you. When you set off on any journey in the future, remember Abraham Lincoln's wise words. In doing so, you'll be able to achieve your weight loss goal much quicker and easier once you begin. Take the time to sharpen your axe. It might just be the difference between success and failure.

Now you understand that failing to prepare is preparing to fail; it's time to begin creating your plan to guarantee success. The first part of planning is to anticipate any barriers that may get in your way. It's essential to consider all potential barriers, not just the clear and obvious ones. Take a moment to think about the next six weeks. Are there any events in the diary or busy days or weeks that may get in your way? These could be birthdays, parties, functions, casual nights out, busy days or times when you're away from home. Then you need to ask yourself, could these affect your results? For some of these situations, the answer may be no, and there's nothing you need to do, but for others, the answer is yes. This is when you must make a plan to overcome these potential barriers.

We all want to have fun and socialise. I'm certainly not going to tell you that you can't celebrate your birthday without a cake or bring in the New Year without a glass of Champagne. Life is for living, enjoying yourself, and socialising with others, and your weight loss journey should be no different. Busy weeks or days can mean you're rushing around, and these are the times when you're more likely to make not-so-smart food choices or skip an exercise session. Suppose these situations can potentially affect your progress or results. In that case, thinking about how you can overcome them before they even happen is crucial. If you do this, you're always one step ahead, allowing you to control the elephant and continue pointing in the correct direction. The way to do this is to write down statements consisting of the actions you will take for your situation.

I will ensure I don't overeat at the party by having a light bite before I go - You may decide to have a healthy light bite before you go to the party. By doing this, you've provided your body with smart food choices, but you've also left a bit of room for some canapés, a slice of cake, or a couple of things from the buffet. Allowing yourself to have some things you enjoy whilst fuelling your body with smart food choices in advance is a great way to stay on track and enjoy the party.

I will say to myself that it is just one day out of 365 - If the party is a big event such as a wedding, Christmas Day, or your birthday, then the first statement isn't going to cut it. Instead, you provide yourself with a day of complete freedom. In doing so, you remain calm at all times and enjoy yourself. When you tell yourself in advance that you can have whatever you want, you will find that you won't overindulge as much as if you go 'F**K it' on the day. By telling yourself it's only one day out of 365, you're looking at the bigger picture rather than feeling like you're sabotaging progress and slipping up. One day is only 0.27% of the year, so it won't make a big dent in your progress if you're taking the correct actions throughout most of the year. This statement prevents the thought of it being a bad day. It encourages the positive feelings of a day to remember. We all have days where we overindulge too much. The vital part is how quickly you get back into the swing of things. Weight loss is a numbers game, and 0.27% of the year will never be a problem, even if you have chocolate for breakfast or copious amounts of alcohol.

I will get back on board straight after a night out - Continuing from the previous statement, after a big night of eating and drinking, it's essential to get back on board as soon as possible. Having a night out of eating and drinking alcohol can quickly increase your calorie intake. This doesn't mean you have to run a marathon the next day to burn them off, but the last thing you want to do is fill day two with not-so-smart food choices and continue loading the body with further calories. By having this statement, you will ensure that you have nutritious meals prepped or even cooked in advance so you can throw them in the microwave or reheat them on the hob and not have to think about what to order from the takeaway. You may not believe me, but a walk in fresh air and a meal made of smart food choices will sort your head out much quicker than a duvet day and takeaway.

I will make twice the amount of food so I can have some in for tomorrow - Batch cooking is a cost-effective way of making your meals, but it is also practical. We all have days where we don't fancy cooking, so it's a good idea to have healthy meals left over from the day before. A night off from the kitchen increases the availability of a quick and nutritious home-cooked meal. Suppose you look at your week and see that you have a busy evening offering a taxi service for your children's extracurricular activities. In that case, healthy leftovers from the night before prevent an unscheduled trip to Captain Cod on the way home.

I will take my lunch with me so I don't have to grab anything whilst I'm out - Many people are out at work all day and pop out to grab something from a local shop or food outlet during their lunch breaks. Even a sandwich can have a scary amount of unnecessary calories due to butter or sauces, so to remain on track, it's best to prepare your lunch at home so you know exactly what's in it. This also helps if you're always rushing around and are tempted by the drive-thru.

I will look at the menu and decide what to eat before I go - Sometimes it's the joy of being out and having a meal cooked for you that's the special part rather than the specific meal you choose. Suppose you're out for a meal with work colleagues, and the occasion doesn't warrant a special meal. In that case, it's a good idea to look at the menu in advance and decide what you will eat before you go out. This will allow you to make a logical decision rather than an irrational one when sitting around the table. It's now compulsory for large food retailers to show calorie content on their menus. Whether you agree with it or not, it's handy for general meals. It's not the best to be reminded how many calories you consume on your birthday, though. Maybe they should offer a birthday menu that doesn't show the calories.

I am going to take my exercise clothes to work so I can go straight to the gym to do a workout - If you plan to go to the gym but find that when you get home each evening, you don't want to go back out, then plan ahead and take your stuff to work. This encourages you to drive directly to the gym, eliminating the barrier of deciding whether to go to the gym or sit on the sofa. By doing this, your workout becomes part of your working day.

I will do a quick workout in the morning - This statement prevents other parts of your day from stopping you from doing a workout. You prioritise a workout by doing it first. Say to yourself that you will do a quick ten-minute workout before you jump in the shower. It will wake you up, and you won't have to think about doing it for the rest of the day. You can get on with your day knowing you've already benefited your health and burnt some calories.

I am going to walk more as I'm sitting at my desk all day - If you have a desk job, which could be a potential barrier as you're mostly sedentary, you can cancel it out by going for a walk at lunchtime. Aim to take a fifteen-minute walk at lunch or park further away from work to get some extra steps in each and every day. Just three thousand additional steps would equate to an extra fifty-four thousand calories burned off that year.

These examples help you create your own statements when you find any potential barriers. Sometimes, there are weeks where you have more than one potential barrier, and it can be challenging to complete actions for all of them. There are other weeks where you would like a big feed. During festive periods and summer holidays, you would like to relax a little with exercise, treat yourself more with not-so-smart food choices, or have a few extra drinks. Your weight loss journey should be easy, but taking more than one action at a time is difficult. Your weight loss journey should be enjoyable and stress-free, so I need to inform you that you don't have to try to lose weight every week.

If you try to lose weight at a time when your life doesn't allow it, you will end up stressed, frustrated and demotivated. You will feel like you can't do it, causing negative emotions to escalate. People who aim to lose weight every week actually do the opposite. They lose weight, gain it, lose it, gain it. Their strive to lose weight in a linear fashion ends up being needles. I always say, what's the point in losing weight if you're going to gain it back? This is why it's always been my purpose to show others how to lose weight and keep it off for good. The first thing to say is that it's unrealistic to lose weight every single week, so don't have those unrealistic expectations.

Weight loss is a case of two steps forward: stop for a chat. You don't have to lose weight every week. When you stop for a chat, you stand still and stay where you are, and that's fine when you're on your weight loss journey. You may lose a few pounds in weeks one and two, but in week three, you have a night out with friends and a couple of kids' parties to attend. Week three shows a few potential barriers on your plan, and it's going to be challenging to lose weight that week. Instead of trying, you decide you will stop for a chat and keep the weight you've lost in weeks one and two off. In doing so, your weight doesn't slide back and forth, you remain calm as you know you're still on track, and you allow yourself to have a good time along the way. This is called a maintenance week.

When planning the next six weeks, you must look at each week to see what you've got on and whether there are any tricky times ahead. For each week, you decide whether it will be a weight loss or maintenance week. A weight loss week is where you've looked and decided that you will 100% be able to lose weight. It's a week where you've not got any potential barriers, or if you do, they are ones you have created an action plan to overcome. They are a week where you can go full throttle and get the number on the scales down as nothing is in your way. If it's looking like a tough week with several potential barriers that will be tricky to overcome, you must label it as a maintenance week. Instead of forcing things, you relax and have a good time with the focus on maintaining your

POINT TO THE DESTINATION

weight. You still take the correct actions, but your objective is to stay the same weight as the previous week. Mapping your weeks out like this makes you much happier and helps you see your weight loss journey in a more realistic and achievable way.

People forget when losing weight that they're in a calorie deficit of around 500 hundred calories each day, which allows them to lose weight. If it's a maintenance week, you have an extra 3500 calories to play with. This can mean skipping an exercise session where you would burn 500 calories or going out for a meal with friends and having a dessert. As long as you don't go over your maintenance calories, you won't gain weight. You don't have to consume all 3500 calories; it's up to this amount.

If you've decided it will be a maintenance week, on Monday morning, do the following…

1. Log into My Fitness Pal.
2. Click on the more tab, and select 'Goal'.
3. Where it says weekly goal, which should be set on losing 0.5-2lb per week, change it to maintain weight. MyFitnessPal will then change your daily calorie goal to maintenance calories.
4. Follow these calorie guidelines for the week

Remember, you don't have to hit this target each day. Depending on your potential barrier and how your week is going, you may consume your usual weight loss calories Monday through Friday to have a blowout at a party over the weekend. This is where it's important to check how you're doing for the week by checking your weekly calories.

If you need to check how many calories you've consumed during the week so far...

1. Log in to MyFitnessPal.
2. Click on the more tab, and select 'Nutrition'.
3. Where it says 'Day View' at the top, change it to 'Week View'.
4. This page will show you the 'Calories Under Weekly Goal'.

Whether it's a weight loss week or a maintenance week, you must track your food intake in MyFitnessPal. By saying it's a weight loss week, you're relaxing your food intake and exercise routine a little. One thing you're not doing is ditching this essential habit when on your weight loss journey. Tracking your food intake ensures you follow the numbers and remain pointing to your destination. The reason why you say it's a maintenance week is so you don't go overboard. Tracking your calories during a maintenance week ensures you don't exceed your allocated 3500 additional calories. Tracking your food intake holds you accountable, keeps you on track, and allows you to adjust. Whatever you do, ensure you track your food intake on MyFitnessPal, whether it's a weight loss or maintenance.

POINT TO THE DESTINATION

Six weeks in advance is always a good time to consider what your life will look like. It gives you sufficient time to search for potential barriers, create action statements to overcome them and decide whether it will be a weight loss or maintenance week. This may not seem like much, but it's your action plan for success. By taking a few minutes at the start of every six-week block, you've mapped out your journey, giving you peace of mind and the confidence you're moving in the right direction. It's simple but highly effective and drastically affects your results and mentality.

Planning ahead keeps you on track and pointing to the destination. You direct the rider and decrease the likelihood of you spooking the elephant. A strong plan is a successful one; without one, you will be unsuccessful. Make sure to think about every possible potential barrier that may get in your way so you can decide what you will do to overcome them. Stress and frustration are key reasons people are unsuccessful on their weight loss journey. By planning ahead, you take this stress out and achieve much more when relaxed. You can see what needs to be done to allow you to stay on track. By anticipating your weeks, you are always one step ahead of any potential barriers. When barriers pop up, you step straight over them as you know what actions to take.

Your To-Do List

1. Anticipate any barriers that could get in your way.
2. Think about what you will do to overcome them.

POINT TO THE DESTINATION

3. Plan your weeks ahead to enable success. Is it a weight loss week or a maintenance week?

PART TWO
PLANNING YOUR MEALS

Planning your journey so you can point to the destination doesn't solely consist of your week and potential barriers. Suppose your food and calorie intake is one of the essential parts of achieving your weight loss goal. In that case, planning your meals is integral to planning your journey. Don't worry; I'm not telling you that you must make a month's worth of meals and put them in sweaty, Spag-bol-stained Tupperware. I am asking you to plan your meals for various reasons. I encouraged you to make smarter food choices in the Grow Yourself chapter. I provided lists of fats, carbohydrates, proteins, vitamins and minerals. You learned which foods were smart food choices and which foods were not-so-smart food choices. I will show you how to make meals from all these foods.

I want you to enjoy your meals, and the only way to ensure this is the case is for you to choose what to eat. It's also the only way you're going to stick to your new way of eating. There's no point in me telling you exactly what to eat as you won't stick to it. With a list of smart food choices and knowing how to plan a meal, you can't go wrong. It gives you the freedom and flexibility to decide what to have for each meal. As long as you aim to consume smart food choices most of the time and track your food intake, you can decide what to eat, and you will be able to keep control of your weight.

The final thing I will teach you in this section is how to eat. I'm not going to start making plane sounds whilst I direct some carrot and swede towards your lips, but I will teach you essential eating habits that will work wonders for your waistline. It's also not the part where I tell you exactly how to eat. I will provide you with a structure for your meals so you can succeed on your weight loss journey. Understanding how to build a meal and planning your daily or weekly meals will help you in many ways. I will show you how to create a meal that provides your body with all the necessary foods to function correctly. Once successfully implemented, you will find this new structure to your way of eating, which won't feel like a diet. Instead, it will feel refreshing, energising, and straightforward.

Planning your meals makes each day decision-free. You are removing the stress of deciding what to eat at each meal. This stress is known as decision paralysis. You don't know what to eat, making mealtime feel like hard work. In the end, you pick a go-to meal you may not benefit from. This is due to the elephant taking over, which can often leave you heading down the wrong road and pointing

POINT TO THE DESTINATION

in the opposite direction. Planning your meals ensures the rider is in control, allowing you to make logical decisions about what to eat to ensure you take the road you aspire to follow. If you sit down for a second and think about your meals, you can select foods from a mixture of food groups, allowing your food intake to be well-balanced. You can plan your meals and weekly food intake to ensure you're consuming smart fats, proteins, carbohydrates, and fruits and vegetables.

In part one, I used the quote, "If I had six hours to chop down a tree, I'd spend the first four hours sharpening the axe." If you plan your meals at the beginning of the week, you will benefit from a stress-free and healthy life and save so much time too. Yes, sitting down and planning your meals will take time initially; however, thoroughly prepared people always save time in the long run. You can reduce trips to the shops each week, cook meals in batches and save time by not having to think about what to eat daily. When you have taken the time to plan your meals, everything will feel more manageable, and the journey towards your weight loss goal will be quicker.

If you don't plan your meals, you start by eating what you want, and that's great as it means you're in control. You eat what you feel like eating every day rather than what you know will help you achieve your goal. When you eat what you feel like eating, you're allowing your emotions and feelings to dictate what you eat. These are six times stronger than your logical thinking, so when presented with the choice of Chicken Salad or Lasagne and Garlic Bread, which do you think will win? There's nothing wrong with a bit of Lasagne and Garlic Bread every once in a while, but when left to make the same choice each day, the not-so-smart foods will win every time.

Not having a plan is taking a punt and hoping for the best. If you want weight loss success, a plan is essential. Without one, thoughts like it's only a couple of biscuits pop into your head to justify your reasoning for unexpectedly eating them. You end up over-consuming not-so-smart and under-consuming smart foods, leading to an unbalanced diet and too many daily calories consumed to lose weight. Your body doesn't work efficiently, your food intake is inconsistent, and it's challenging to see sustainable weight loss. You're left scratching your head and wondering why things aren't working for you. You then try to justify your failures by stating that tracking your calories doesn't work and decide a silly diet is the solution, which we all know is a ridiculous idea. All along, you've been inconsistently logging your food and drink consumption as you've just been eating what you feel like and only tracking when you consume smart foods.

You already know how many calories you should be consuming to lose or maintain weight, but I need to show you how much you should be eating in terms of volume. Throughout this book, you're discovering a way of eating that will work long-term, not only during your weight loss journey but for the rest of your life. The term 'balanced diet' is always mentioned, and most people know that it means consuming sufficient fats, carbohydrates, proteins, vitamins, and minerals; they don't know how much they should aim to consume of each. I'm not informing you to begin measuring and weighing each food you add to your meals. Although accurate logging would take place, it's just not practical. A taller person requires more food than a shorter person, and all humans come attached with their very own set of measuring tools that are specific to them. The set of measuring tools I'm talking about are your hands. A taller person would have larger hands than a smaller person. Therefore, the serving size of each food group will be the correct amount for each individual. You know to consume more smart fats, proteins, carbohydrates, and a rainbow of fruits and vegetables. Now, look at how many of these smart foods you should consume each meal.

Protein Serving—One Palm-Sized Portion - Each meal should consist of one palm-sized serving from the smart proteins column.

Vegetables/Salad Serving—Two Handful Sized Portions - Once you've selected your choice of smart protein, add two fist-sized portions of salad or vegetables to ensure you consume plenty of vitamins and minerals. A handful-sized portion is grabbing your vegetables or salad. This big serving will also fill your plate with low-calorie, high-volume food.

Carbohydrates serving- One Cupped Hand Portion - Next, pour smart carbohydrates into the palm of your hand. A serving is the amount that fits in one cupped hand. If you're ever cooking for other people, place your carbohydrate serving in its own pan to ensure the correct serving for you.

Fats serving - One thumb-sized portion - Finally, to create a balanced meal, select a smart fat and cut the amount that's the size of your thumb off. Obviously, this doesn't work with all fats, such as olive oil, but it does give you a guideline of the size of smart fats. If it's a liquid, it would need to be measured out. One serving of smart fats in liquid form is 15ml.

Each meal you consume doesn't have to be perfectly balanced in the way I've just explained. In a perfect world, the above is what you would consume, but it's unrealistic, and we don't live in one. A typical day consists of three meals: breakfast, lunch, and dinner. If you are recommended to consume one palm-sized serving per meal, that would be three palm-sized portions per day. How and when you decide to consume them is your decision. This is why I've outlined the volumes per day below instead.

Protein Serving Per Day - Three Palm-Sized Portions
Vegetables/Salad Per Day - Six Handful Sized Portions
Carbohydrates Per Day - Three Cupped Hand Portions
Fats Per Day - Three Thumb-Sized Portions

If you do this daily, you will provide your body with everything it needs. You will feel satisfied with your meals, energised each day, and keep illness and disease away. If you're left thinking there's no way on earth you can have that amount of food, you don't have to; these are guidelines. Being smart isn't solely about consuming nutritious foods; it's gaining smart skills too. Smart skills may not seem much, but if you practice them, they will prove to be extremely valuable. Some refer to smart skills as mindful eating, meaning using all of your physical and emotional senses to experience and enjoy food. Mindful eating increases gratitude for food, helps you identify hunger and fullness cues, and improves the overall eating experience.

The first smart skill you must acquire is identifying your hunger cues. This is when the hunger hormone ghrelin kicks in, which is the appropriate time to eat. More often than not, we eat for other reasons related to our emotions and habits. You nip into the kitchen because you're bored, eat comfort foods when sad, and grab food from a food outlet as it's a habit you've settled into over time. The first thing you must do before consuming a meal or snack is to get into the habit of drinking a glass of water. This will ensure you remain hydrated, which is good, but it will also take up space in the stomach, reducing hunger. A person may think they are hungry when they are actually thirsty, so it's always a good idea to check it's not the latter. Water contains zero calories, but the food you eat for mistaking hunger for thirst could be in the hundreds. A simple and smart skill to control your calorie intake and, therefore, your weight is to drink water each time you think you're hungry.

Once you've allowed a short amount of time to see if it was water your body has been crying out for, you must ask yourself, "Am I hungry?". If you are still hungry after your glass of water, it's clearly hunger, and it's time to eat. If you find that you're not as hungry as you initially thought before drinking, it was thirst, meaning you don't need to eat. Asking yourself if you're hungry encourages your mind and body to become in tune with one another. If you ask, it will tell you. However, most people don't stop to ask or think before they take the action of reaching into the cupboards. If the body has confirmed that it requires feeding, you must ask yourself, "Does my body need this?". This question encourages you to stop and think about what you're putting in your body. Are you providing it with the nutrients it needs, or are you providing it with not-so-smart food choices? The smart skill of asking yourself whether you're hungry and what your body asks for allows reflection, time, and confirmation. You stop to think whether you're eating for the right reasons and decide whether the foods you consume will help or hinder progress. Asking yourself how you feel will prevent emotional eating and promote only eating when physically hungry.

'Hara hachi bun me' is a Japanese phrase that translates to "Eat until you are eight parts (out of ten) full" or "Belly 80% full". This is thought to delay the stomach stretch receptors that help signal satiety. Eating until you're full would cause a constant stretching of the stomach, increasing the amount of food needed to feel full. Similar practices can also be found in China and India. I find the Indian phrase "You should fill one-third of the stomach with liquid, another third with food, and leave the rest empty." a relevant one. It confirms the view to drink fluids before eating, and this dates back to 400 BC and shows that you don't need to reinvent the wheel. Instead, replicate and clone the success of the people before us. Bright spots can also be found in history books. The third smart skill is to "Eat until you're satisfied rather than full", which is the same as 'Hara hachi bun me'. Once you've identified your physical hunger and have decided to consume smart foods, you must acquire the habit of stopping once you're satisfied rather than full to prevent the stomach from stretching. Over time, your stomach will be satisfied with smaller quantities, leading to better body weight control. If you leave food on your plate regularly and don't want it to go to waste, decrease your portion size the next time you eat.

When consuming a meal, a couple of smart skills will help you identify when you're satisfied rather than full. More often than not, we eat too quickly and without paying full attention to what we're eating. This can be grabbing something before rushing to work in the morning or shoving your sandwich in as quickly as possible before going into the next meeting. Doing this prevents the body from mentally processing what you're eating, causing more food to be consumed before it has decided it's satisfied rather than full. We've all had a big dinner and then felt stuffed afterwards. We've got it into the body so quickly that it hasn't had time to process the sheer volume of the Sunday Roast.

Another common scenario is eating food without paying full attention to what we're eating. Many people eat their meals in front of the TV, causing them to pay more attention to the latest series than the meal in front of them.

The same goes for watching a film with some snacks. You're so engrossed in the movie that you've missed your satisfied cues. You don't feel sick because of the gore in the film but the volume of chocolate you've consumed. Smart skills four and five prevent these situations from occurring. When consuming any food, consciously decide to eat slowly and without distractions. This means putting your knife and fork down and having a conversation with family, sitting at the table without the TV on, and not eating at your desk or in the car. These two smart skills will prevent overeating and allow your body to mentally process the foods you're consuming.

Smart skills recap

- Drink a glass of water before you eat.
- Ask yourself if you're hungry and whether your body needs the food you're about to consume.
- Eat until you're satisfied rather than full. Hara hachi bun me. Eat until you're 80% full.
- Eat slowly
- Eat without distractions

What meal are you going to work on first?

You should now see how your meals are starting to take shape. Tracking your calories ensures you lose and keep control of your weight. Consuming smart foods provides the body with the nutrients it needs to feel energised and function correctly. Planning your meals ensures the rider is in control, preventing emotional eating. Following the food portion guidelines ensures you consume the correct amount of each food group and prevents overeating. Smart food skills create healthy eating habits to allow the body to identify genuine hunger cues, prevent the stomach from stretching, and enable the mind to process the foods you've consumed. All these actions come together to make controlling your weight easier and automated. When this happens, you won't have to track your calories every single day. You won't have to check your lists of smart and not-so-smart foods. You won't have to think about your smart skills as you will automatically do them. You won't have to look at your hands every time you measure food. You have to learn these things now so you don't have to think about them in the future.

All of us have bright spots with regard to our eating habits and food intake. It's your job to investigate and clone these bright spots to allow success in other areas. Please take a minute to look through your daily food intake on MyFitnessPal. What are you currently doing well? Is it a particular meal or a specific day of the week? Where are you consuming smart foods? Which meals contain the appropriate calories? Which meals are you in control of?

Then, it would help if you found the days or meals where you could clone your bright spots to have full control over all meals. Take a moment to think about which part of your eating routine needs improving. Is there a particular meal where your calorie intake is way too high? Is there a meal that's made up of uncontrolled portions? Does your breakfast contain no colours of the rainbow? It could be your unscheduled snacking. Or are you eating your lunch in a rush?

You know the importance of taking things one step at a time. To shrink the change and script the critical moves. This is why you should only aim to change one meal at a time. Remember to make the moves that count, the critical moves that will make the most significant change to your eating routine. Which part of your eating routine will you change at which mealtime?

How do you plan the week?

The key to successful weight loss is planning ahead, and the same goes for planning your meals. Planning takes a minimal amount of time yet dramatically impacts the quality of your weeks. This is why you must plan your eating routine at the beginning of each week. Begin by looking at your weekly schedule, so you know what you have coming up. If you have a busy couple of days mid-week, decide if you're going to cook a few extra meals up before so you can reheat and remain on track. If you have an event over the weekend where your calories will be higher than usual, work out how many calories you need to reduce each other day to balance the numbers so you can remain under your weekly total calories. Plan ahead with your meals based on what you have on that week.

Once you've examined ways to overcome any potential barriers, it's time to look at each meal. We are creatures of habit, meaning we eat similar breakfasts and lunches daily. Look at your lists of smart foods and decide which food from each food group will feature in your breakfasts. Then, do the same for your lunches and dinners. If you find an imbalance in a meal, such as smart carbohydrates for breakfast consisting of porridge and blueberries, prioritise smart fats and smart proteins in the other meals. Each meal will be different. It's your job to plan your meals in advance to ensure you consume all the foods your body needs.

This chapter has informed you how to plan your meals and has provided guidelines for measuring portions of each food group. What you eat is important, but more importantly, eat what works for you. This is a gentle reminder. If you try to eat meals you feel you should be eating or eat foods you think you have to eat, you aren't going to stick with it. You don't have to fit in and copy what everybody else is eating. Instead, thinking of a way of eating that works for you would be best. You don't have to eat something if you don't like it, but try new things gradually, and you never know, that may change. Planning your own meals rather than following somebody else's diet plan allows you to be in control. This may sound scary, but by now, you've been provided with all of the tools needed to plan your meals in a way that will work for you.

Your To-Do List

1. Look at your current portion sizes. How do they compare to the suggested serving sizes I mentioned earlier?

2. Pick the first meal of the day to work on. Which meal or day are you going to improve first.
3. Sit down and take a moment to plan your meals for the week. While doing this, it's best to look at your planning ahead worksheet to identify potential barriers.

11

SHAPE THE ROAD

PART ONE
TWEAK THE ENVIRONMENT

Shaping the road is the final thing to do to make your weight loss journey effortless. Planning your journey ensures it's smooth without any bumps along the way. Shape the Road is cutting back any overgrown branches that may scratch the elephant or the rider during the journey. Shaping the road encourages you to focus on the surrounding environment, making change even more straightforward by removing friction from the trail. Two things are needed to shape the road —Tweak The Environment and Build New Habits. We attribute people's behaviours to who they are rather than their situation. The

SHAPE THE ROAD

environments we are in shape us into behaviours that help or hinder progress. Tweaking the environment makes the right behaviours easier and the wrong behaviours harder. If you want to change things, you must pay close attention to social signals, as they can either guarantee a change effort or prevent it from happening. The second part of Shape The Road is building new habits. Once a behaviour is habitual, it's free and doesn't tax the rider. Change is easy when positive habits are automated, requiring no extra effort. For anything to change, the rider has to start acting differently. To change your behaviour, you've got to change the situation you're in. This is done by shaping the road you're about to follow.

Each former chapter has gradually helped you map out your journey. The road is straight and the directions are clear. Tweak the environment is everything surrounding you or affecting you on your journey. This includes the people around you, what's in the kitchen cupboards, and your sleep pattern. Looking at these areas allows a smooth journey and prevents tough decisions or tricky situations. It is always best to avoid conflict, and tweaking the environment, especially concerning people, prevents issues with loved ones that may cause frustration. We all make bad decisions, but the key to success is to prevent and restrict as many of those bad decisions as possible. Some slip through the net; however, the idea of tweaking the environment is to reduce them as much as possible by preventing tough decisions from being made.

It may get tricky if you set off to lose weight without tweaking the environment. Tricky times mean uncertain

SHAPE THE ROAD

times, leading to unpredictable weight fluctuations. This can cause you to get frustrated with either yourself or the people around you. Reason six for thinking weight loss is hard is being too hard on yourself. When you do this, your enthusiasm and positivity can be sapped out of you, creating reason ten why you believe weight loss is hard: You're exhausted trying to lose weight. Not to forget reason nine, it's not you; it's the situation you're in. By tweaking the environment, you eliminate these three reasons why you believe weight loss is hard. You will still lose weight if you stop reading this book right now, but you might as well avoid any issues and uncertain times by tweaking the environment to make weight loss easier.

Stop for a second and ask yourself: Am I giving myself the best chance of success? Take some time to look at yourself and see the future. What do you see around you? Does the environment give you the best chance of success? Tweaking the environment begins with what you see. The first place I wish for you to start is by asking yourself— Am I surrounded by positive people? I'm starting with this because it's such a common issue. Humans are social creatures, and we take cues from those around us. We are naturally biased towards wanting to be part of a common social structure, meaning we end up fitting in with our friends and family.

We like what they like, and we do what they do. We think like they think and behave as they behave. Now, you may have gone against the grain and decided you want to lose weight. You may even be the only person you know who wants to lose weight. It could be the first time you're venturing off on a journey alone. It's like deciding to run a marathon. Your friends and family may not want to do it, but to be successful, you need some cheerleaders along the way.

The people you spend the most time with shape who you are. They determine which conversations dominate your attention, how you feel, and which direction you head in. The people you associate with determine as much as 95% of your success or failure in life. That's huge. The dream in your heart may be bigger than the environment you find yourself in. Sometimes, you need to get out of that environment to see your dream fulfilled.

Don't worry; I'm not telling you to ditch everyone. I'm not telling you that you need to stop speaking to your friends and family or quit your job. Getting out of the environment doesn't mean you need to leave everyone you've loved or known behind. But if you find they're not helping you, you need to tweak the environment by rallying the herd and getting them on your side. This way, you create positive feelings around you whilst ensuring no one is holding you back.

Behaviour is contagious, and rallying the herd ensures that contagious behaviour is positive, as the people around you are on your side. I want you to think about who you spend the most time with. Think of five to ten people — Are they work colleagues? Are they friends of yours? Or are they all family members? Are they your biggest supporters in life? Will they do anything to ensure you succeed on your weight loss journey? Or will they try and get you to give up and sabotage your progress because they're not trying to lose weight themselves, and you're showing them up? You are the average of the five to ten people you spend the most time with. Who's in your herd?

Rallying the herd builds a support structure around you, and it's time for you to create your own. It all starts with the five to ten people you spend the most time with. It's important to have them on board. How could you tweak your relationships to ensure they're supportive and not sabotaging your progress? Some friends, family, and colleagues are good influences; others like to upset the apple cart. Instead of socialising over a drink or food, think about how you could have fun with friends more actively. What activities could you do together that will help you lose weight?

Communities of like-minded people on a similar weight loss journey can be worth their weight in gold. These can be in-person with friends or on social media in weight loss groups. Swapping tips, sharing moments, and helping each other are fantastic ways to know you're not alone. Which communities could you join to help support you throughout your journey?

Building a support structure within your home, social group, and community will strengthen your network and make your journey fun, supportive, and successful. How could you ensure everyone is on board with your weight loss journey?

If your current herd isn't helping, you have one of two options. The first is to bring in other people, as any journey alone will be a tough one. It's always good to surround yourself with people going through the same thing as you, people trying to lose weight too, and those on the same journey as you. Ideally, you are surrounding yourself with people who are losing weight in a sensible and smart way rather than crash dieting. Get in touch with that friend who likes country walks. Speak to the person in the office who brings healthy lunches to work. Get in touch with the relative who has lost weight and managed to keep it off. Surround yourself with people going through the same thing as you. These are the people who get it. Spending more time with these people will ensure your herd is supportive.

The other option, which can be done in tangent with option one, will be to have a conversation with those around you. You don't need to call a village meeting; however, if your best friend, partner, or parents aren't supporting you, you must address this thorn in your side. Even though, they're being a pain in the backside, you must ensure you do it in a way that doesn't rub them up the wrong way. If it rubs them up the wrong way, you're just going to be faced with more resistance. Start by telling them why you want to lose weight. If your 'why' is strong enough, it should be strong enough for them to want to help you. Step two is where you ask if they can help you. If the answer is yes, tell them how they can help you. This could be by being more positive and supportive around you, changing how you socialise with them, or holding you accountable. Once you've explained what they can do, come to an agreement and outline how they will help you. Whatever you do, don't tell them to stop doing something. People don't like that. You can't change people. All you can change is how you react to them and what you do with them.

When tweaking the environment, the next area to consider is ensuring you get enough sleep. I don't want to be one of those nagging people who tell you to go to bed earlier, but it's the most important thing for your health and plays a crucial role in weight management. Not getting sufficient sleep prevents your batteries from being recharged overnight, causing you to run at 75% during the day. Due to this deprivation, you wake up feeling tired. You're like an old iPhone trying to run on the latest update. To try and keep up with the day, you search for energy from food to make up the 25% you should've received from an extra two hours of sleep. When the body requires energy, it demands it in the simplest forms to allow an energy boost as quickly as possible. This means the need for sugar, meaning not-so-smart foods are consumed. A 25% sleep deprivation leads to a 25% increase in calories consumed.

Sleep is the best way for your body to re-energise. When you get sufficient sleep each evening, you will find an improvement in your food choices and a reduction in the amount of calories your body tells you to consume. Smart food choices packed full of energy and nutrients will be consumed, causing you to feel fresh, healthy, and ready to take on your day. The feeling of being energised and running at 100% allows you to feel as though you have the energy to perform an exercise session. When you complete a workout, you feel more productive and happier and gain a further energy boost without consuming any calories. Exercise increases your energy levels throughout each day, but it also helps you to sleep better. With a little work, you can see the positive effects of getting sufficient sleep. I encourage you to tweak your sleep pattern, particularly your sleep routine. It is the foundation of self-care.

It's not just the duration of how long you sleep; it's the quality too. Like food, the quality affects how you feel and greatly benefits the body. This is why it's important to follow a sleep routine when the countdown to bedtime begins. Begin by shutting down. Select a time when you stop checking your phone or doing work. You don't want to be doing anything that mentally stimulates you so close to bedtime. Aim to begin shutting down at a similar time each evening, as the body loves routine. Once you've eliminated the stressors that stimulate you throughout the day, it's time to relax. Relaxing before bed slows the mind and body down. You want a clear separation of night and day to avoid taking the busy day to bed with you. Take a bath or shower before bed, do a ten-minute yoga session or read a book. Make your bedroom something you can't wait to get into. Soft pillows and comfy pyjamas are a great place to start. Use soft lighting in the run-up before bed to allow melatonin secretion to begin. Light scented candles, turn on aroma diffusers thirty minutes before bed and let essential oils calm and prepare you for sleep.

Some of the bedtime recommendations sound like the obvious parts of relaxing and going to sleep. However, we dismiss these actions as we would rather watch another episode of a series, scroll through social media, or have a bottle of wine. These three things might seem like switching off, yet they actually stimulate the mind and decrease the quality of your sleep. Improve the duration and quality of your sleep, and you will find weight management will be easier, and your health will improve. You will also have control over how many calories you consume daily. Begin with the duration and then look at tweaking the environment to enhance the quality. Everything doesn't have to be changed at once. You don't need whale music, a mud mask, and a foot spa on day one. Although it does sound tempting, doesn't it?

You've thought about your bedtime routine and who's supporting you; the final thing to cover regarding tweaking the environment is what's in the house. Your house should be your safe space. It's where the battle is won, which is why your home needs to help you lose weight, eat well and remain active. Unfortunately, many homes are sucking them into time spent gaining weight, eating poorly and remaining inactive. This is why the third and final part of tweaking the environment is tweaking your home. Your home tweaks include improving the kitchen, setting up your workout space, and making your home a positive environment. These tweaks will ensure you live in a home that's on your side.

The first thing to do is look at what's in the kitchen. You're now kitted out with the lists of smart and no-so-smart foods. It's time to do a kitchen MOT and check various parts of your kitchen. When you venture into your kitchen, is it one full of temptation or one that encourages you to eat healthy foods and stay on track?

SHAPE THE ROAD

The first part of your kitchen MOT is to check what's in the cupboards. With your list of smart and not-so-smart foods, check each kitchen cupboard individually to see what your kitchen is made up of. Remember, not-so-smart foods are allowed, so you don't need to chuck all of them in the bin. However, if your kitchen is made up predominantly of not-so-smart foods, some of them have to go. Your goal for weight control is to consume 80% of your calorie intake from smart foods and 20% from not-so-smart food choices. The foods in your kitchen cupboards should match or be similar to these percentages. This way, you're ensuring you have smart foods readily available and not-so-smart foods not so much. The kitchen MOT also applies to your fridge and freezer space too. Work your way around the kitchen to see what's in your cupboards.

Once you've discovered what's in your kitchen cupboards and have cleared out some not-so-smart items to balance the kitchen cupboards, it's important to look at who does the shopping. It doesn't matter what it is; everything brought into the house will be eaten eventually, so you need to control what comes into your home. The only way to ensure your kitchen is full of the smart foods you should be consuming is to ensure you do the food shop. This way, you can plan your weekly meals and buy the appropriate foods. If you find that your partner or parents do the food shop, you can't allow them to do it for you. You have to do your own shopping. Hopefully, they will allow you to take control of your home's food intake. If they don't, things may be a little tricky. If this happens, you must leave them to it and do your own food shop and follow your own meals. Once they see how delicious yours are and see your amazing results, they will be asking you to shop and cook for them too.

You now have control over the kitchen; the final check on your kitchen MOT is to decide what needs to be more visible. Every time you decide you're hungry, you must be faced with smart foods. They should be staring at you on the kitchen sides, be at the front on the fridge shelves, and featured like trophies in your cupboards. Fruit needs to be featured in your fruit bowl, vegetables need to be fresh and ready in the fridge, and your porridge oats on the side in some fancy containers. If you have children, hopefully, you will provide them with smart foods too. If they like packs of crisps or chocolate bars, try making them less visible. Place them all in a specific cupboard so you aren't tempted each time you open the cupboards to get your smart foods out. Make smart foods more visible and not-so-smart foods less visible.

A home should be an active one, regardless of whether you've decided to be more active in or outside of the house. If it has been raining, you need a space to do your squats or a ten-minute workout. In your home, take a look around and decide where to set up a space to workout. This space will be home to your dumbbells, exercise mat, and sweat towel. It needs to be visible to you and readily available. This removes any potential barrier to participation and keeps a visual reminder to be active in place. If you've decided to increase your activity levels with your children, a football or netball net in your garden might

SHAPE THE ROAD

be a visual reminder to get outside and enjoy some active family time. Take a moment to think about how you can make your home an active one.

The final part of tweaking your home is to make it a positive one. You've created a house of cheerleaders by creating a support structure around you and having the people you live with on your side. The changes to your sleep routine, kitchen cupboards, and workout space ooze positive thoughts and feelings. In the Find The Feeling chapter, I encouraged you to create visual reminders of both your progress and where you're heading. If you've decided to set up the pound coin jars, place them in a clear position. If you've decided to hang up an item of clothing you can't wait to wear, go and hang it up immediately. Place the photo of your holiday destination on the fridge door. Ensure you're reminded daily of why you're doing this. All of these minor tweaks come together to transform your home, giving you the best chance of success.

You will still be able to lose weight without tweaking the environment, but it will be even easier if you do. Get out there and make succeeding on your weight loss journey even more effortless. I've covered a variety of areas that could be tweaked. It's important to remember the messages from previous chapters. Focus on one change at a time. You don't need to rush off and change everything immediately. If areas need to be tweaked, add them to your list of possible changes you could make. If a change is a critical move, add it to your list of critical moves and place it in order of most critical. The change you must focus on first is the most critical. Which change is the most important? Decide what it is and always make this change first.

Your To-Do List

1. The first is to ask yourself what needs to be tweaked — Which environmental changes will make things easier?
2. Think about who you need to talk to — Who do you need to inform about your desires and ambitions?
3. Think about the most critical tweaks to be made — Is it clearing out the house, setting up your workout space, or sorting out your sleep pattern? Ask yourself which tweaks are the most important to you.

PART TWO
BUILDING NEW HABITS

Now that you've started to tweak the environment and rally the herd, you've begun to shape the road. You've cut away branches that may scrape the elephant or rider along their journey. Building new habits helps you shape the road even more, but more importantly, puts this ride in cruise control. Any person who maintains the same weight will have automated healthy habits. If you can put your weight loss journey in cruise control, you won't have to worry about gaining weight ever again. You're already beginning your journey in cruise control by creating your roadmap. You will get into the habit of tracking your food intake, eating smarter, scripting your critical moves, and planning your weeks and meals. These changes are new habits, but you must also learn how to build new habits too.

If you put this ride in cruise control, you won't have to stop and think about what to do. You'll just do it. If there's ever an opportunity to remove a decision, take it, as you can only make a certain amount of decisions each day. The more decisions you make, the more mistakes you make. The last thing you should do is decide what to eat when hungry. You don't want to be thinking about whether you should be exercising. You should do it without even thinking about it. Building new habits allows you to create automated healthy ones, putting your journey in cruise control.

New habits may be tedious because they are a tool to help you achieve your goal rather than the emotion of joy when you step on the scales. They teach you how to be a good rider on your journey, helping you lose weight and keep it off forever. Building new habits improves the overall quality of your life and results. They allow you to thrive rather than solely survive. If you ever take a break from losing weight, new habits will keep you where you are, allowing you to pick up where you left off. New habits create longevity. They enable you to remain at your target weight for the rest of your life.

You've done all the hard work (in our case, the easy work) and have successfully reached your target weight. You feel ecstatic and run around celebrating, and so you should. But, and this is a big but, which can lead to a bigger butt. You stop making changes as you've hit your target weight and have decided you don't need to do anything else. It's time to reap the rewards and enjoy yourself. You resort back to the old habits you acquired over your lifetime. Due to this, you gain back all the weight you've lost. I'm sure this has happened to you in the past. Building new habits is essential when making sure weight gain never happens again. When this happens, you have control of your weight and never have to try and lose weight ever again.

Before you build new habits, you must examine whether your current habits are helping or hindering your progress. Habits that help and habits that hinder are the same in how they work. The difference is habits that help feel bland at the moment but provide compounded benefits over time. Hindering habits are pleasurable at the moment but compound negatively and cause weight gain over time. Which direction are your current habits taking you in?

If you discover you have a habit that's hindering and steering you in the wrong direction, you must notice and name it. Don't sweat about it; building new habits will reduce these hindering habits. When you notice you're doing something, such as sneaking into the treat cupboard during the ad breaks or driving home instead of the gym, call yourself out on it. Hold yourself accountable.

Key points when building new habits

Forget the hindering habits - It's important to notice and name them, but don't worry about them. There's no point using your energy on these hindering habits, just like I told you not to worry about the 'not-so-smart 'foods in your diet. Instead, it would be best to focus on new and beneficial habits. Remember your bright spots and always focus on what you're doing well; this strengthens the growth mindset. Spending your time focusing on the hindering habits is a fixed mindset issue. When you focus on the beneficial actions, the hindering habits will slowly begin to disappear. When you do this, the pressure is taken off, and you follow the road of least resistance and continue on a journey of self-improvement.

Shrink the change - New habits will be ones that will be around for the rest of your life so there's no rush to change everything. You don't have to master them overnight. You also don't need to make big changes. Instead, start small and simple. Remember, the more complicated a task is, the more likely a person will fail. You must shrink the change to ensure your new habits are so easy to fulfil that you can't say no. When you do this, the elephant isn't spooked, as it doesn't need any motivation to do it. The easier it is, the more consistent you will be, meaning you've created a new, beneficial habit, as habits are created by doing the same thing repeatedly. There's nothing impressive about doing a difficult task once. What's impressive is sticking with the same task time and time again, regardless of difficulty. Your objective is to remain at least 80% consistent with each action to begin making it a habit. To do this, you need to shrink the change.

Gradually build it up - When you start with a small change, you allow time to master the task and remain consistent with the habit. Think of it like levels or grades. You don't become a black belt on day one or head off to University at age four. Habits should be treated the same. Each week, month, or even year, you evolve and gradually build up your actions to allow further improvement. You have plenty of time to build things up. The key is consistency. When you gradually build new habits, your changes will feel effortless, willpower will increase, and any change you make will stick.

How to build beneficial habits

The following four steps are from James Clear, author of Atomic Habits: Tiny Changes, Remarkable Results. I highly recommend his book. Follow these four steps when creating new habits.

Make it as obvious as possible - The first thing to do is to make it as obvious as possible. An example is creating a statement to commit to, e.g. "As soon as I wake up, I will stretch for five minutes by the side of my bed.". This is obvious because it's the first thing you do once your feet hit the floor. You've also said you will do it by the side of your bed, avoiding any distractions of the day coming your way. You can make it even more obvious by setting your alarm to say, "Wake up, it's stretch time". You could place this statement in a mini photo frame and position it by your bedside. If you plan to exercise in the morning, make your intentions obvious and put your workout gear and trainers out as an obvious reminder when you wake up. If a new habit is to eat an omelette each morning for breakfast, place the eggs on the kitchen worktops.

Make it attractive - Once you've thought about how to make it obvious, you need to think how to make it attractive. The more attractive an opportunity is, the more likely it is to become habit-forming. The easiest way to think of this is how a dog learns new tricks. You make it do something you want and reward it with a treat or tennis ball. As time passes, you no longer need the reward, as it creates a new habit. Ask yourself — How can you make a new habit so attractive you can't wait to do it? Let's say you want to watch a thirty-minute episode of your favourite series. You can tell yourself, "Before I sit down to watch an episode, I will do twenty jumping squats". This combines a task with a reward. You need to exercise but want to watch your favourite TV show. If you binge-watch more episodes, that's fine because you've managed to do eighty jumping squats and have been rewarded for it.

Make it easy - The next thing you need to work on is making your new habit as easy as possible. You know the importance of shrinking the change, which you must do when forming new habits. The easiest way is to decrease the task so much that you don't even notice it. If you aren't currently exercising, begin with five minutes. If you want to do some squats, start with five repetitions. If you want to eat vegetables, begin with one broccoli head on your plate. There's plenty of time for you to build this up in the future. The key here is to get you to create a new healthy habit you can be consistent with. Always begin with an action you can do; don't feel it needs to be complicated. Focus on taking small actions that compound to deliver big results. The amount of time you have been performing habits is not as important as the number of times you've performed it. Small and regular are better than big and infrequent. How can you make a new habit as easy as possible so you go and do it?

SHAPE THE ROAD

Make it satisfying - The final thing needed when building a new habit is to make it immediately satisfying. We are more likely to repeat the behaviour when the experience is immediately satisfying. If you need to exercise, set up a chart on your fridge where you can tick off an exercise session. Just seeing the ticks add up makes it immediately satisfying. If you want to make your lunches at home rather than buying them from a shop, set up a money pot. Every time you make lunch, immediately place the money you saved by making your lunch into that pot. This makes it satisfying every day as you see small amounts of cash build up in your pot. You can then use this money to buy a new outfit or use it towards a family holiday once you've hit your weight loss goal. To get the habit to stick, you need to feel immediately satisfied, even if it's in a small way. What's immediately rewarded is repeated.

Habit Stacking

New habits are created by making them obvious, attractive, easy, and satisfying. The easiest way to stick with your new habits day in and day out is to stack your habits up. Think about which habit you wish to introduce to your daily routine first. It can be anything that will help you move closer towards your weight loss goal. Remember, it needs to be a small habit that takes, at most, five minutes to complete. It also needs to be something you can be at least 80% consistent with. If you can't be over 80% consistent, shrink the change. To allow yourself to be as consistent as possible, stack it on top of a current one you're already consistently doing. A habit like brushing your teeth, taking a shower, boiling the kettle, or even walking through the front door. Something already automated and in cruise control is the best place to start. This way, you will automatically do your new habit before, during, or after your current habit, making it easy to stick to.

Once you've remained consistent with your new habit and stacked it onto a current one, you can stack up another. If you decide to do ten squats every time you boil the kettle and are consistent with this new habit, stack an additional ten press-ups on top of it. A simple and automated task, such as boiling the kettle, becomes an opportunity to be more active, healthier and tone up, without taking any time out of your day. Let's take a look at what your habit stack may look like.

1. It's time for dinner, and I throw my chicken in the oven.
2. After I throw my chicken in the oven, I chop up my vegetables.
3. After I chop up my vegetables, I will do five minutes of aerobic exercise.
4. After five minutes of aerobic exercise, I will do five minutes of resistance training.
5. After five minutes of resistance training, I will sit at the table and enjoy my meal.
6. After finishing my meal, I will go for a ten-minute walk.

As you can see, you start by beginning to make your dinner. You do this every day, which is why it's an excellent current habit to start stacking things on top of. You then move on to cutting up vegetables, which is the first of your new habits to ensure you eat more colours of the rainbow. Once you're consistent with this habit each dinner time, you stack the second new habit on top. Once your food prep is done, you have ten minutes to spare until your chicken is ready to take out of the oven. Due to this, you decide to stack a second new habit of doing five minutes of aerobic exercise. Remember, although you have ten minutes available, a new habit should never be longer than five minutes.

Once this habit is consistently stacked to your dinner routine, you stack an additional five minutes of resistance training onto your aerobic exercise and choose to do one set of press-ups, squats and sit-ups. These three new habits allow you to eat more vegetables, improve your fitness, and tone your body. The spare ten minutes are filled, and it's dinner time. You take the chicken out of the oven and sit at the table. Sitting at a table without distractions is your fourth new habit and teaches you to eat more mindfully.

Finally, after remaining consistent with your new dinner routine for a few months, you decide to go for a ten-minute walk after your evening meal. Before you know it, you're sufficiently active, and it's not taking much extra time. If you have kids, get them involved in this evening routine too. See everything as an opportunity rather than a potential barrier. That's what someone with a growth mindset would do.

Habits are, in essence, behavioural autopilot. They allow lots of good behaviours to happen without the rider taking charge. Remember, the rider's self-control is exhaustible, so it's a huge plus if many positive actions can happen for free on autopilot. Habit stacking works best when the cue is highly specific and immediately actionable. The cue must be a specific action rather than a general one for it to work. Think kettle boiling, phone pinging, walking through the front door, or your alarm going off. You also need to make sure you can be consistent with your new habits. They must be so small you can remain at least 80% consistent with it. Shrink it so small that it can be quickly done in less than five minutes. Only stack a second habit once you've managed to be consistent with your first for at least two weeks. Whatever you do, don't rush this. New habits take time to be consistent with. You don't want to shock the elephant with too much change at once.

Your To-Do List

1. Pick a new habit you wish to include — What new habit would help you lose weight and keep it off?
2. Build your new habit up — How do you plan on making this new habit obvious, attractive, easy, and satisfying?
3. Start stacking your habits over time — Which current habit could you begin to stack new ones on

SHAPE THE ROAD

top of? Plan your weeks ahead to enable success. Is it a weight loss week or a maintenance week?

12

RIDE INTO THE SUNSET

You've shaped the road you're about to follow by tweaking the environment and building new habits. You should now see how you're going to keep the weight off. You've planned everything you need to do week by week and learned everything you need to know about weight loss, meaning there are no more doubts in your mind or information overload. It can be extremely easy to overlook the true power of shrinking the change, following your bright spots, and smoothing the road; however, we make the biggest mistakes in these areas. A lot of effort goes into starting your weight loss journey, which initially helps you lose weight. However, if you're still acting the same way in the same environment, you won't be able to keep the weight off. No matter how compelling the vision is, there are still obstacles in the way. Whatever you do, don't overlook these essential parts.

Make sure the road is clear so you can move down it without any issues. The road is never-ending. It's an ongoing project. Don't feel overwhelmed or scared by this, as your new habits will become automated. The fact that there is no end should feel great as it means you don't have to do everything all at once. You can take things easy as you don't need to rush, allowing you to enjoy the journey by making gradual changes to your current lifestyle. Build new habits and stack them on top of one another over time. This is a journey of self-improvement where you must keep asking yourself — How can I keep improving my lifestyle and continue down this road?

You've officially completed the main chapters in this book, meaning that you've planned everything you need to plan and learned everything you need to learn, but don't rush off just yet. I know you're keen to begin; however, there are a few more things left for you to do before you ride off into the sunset. You need to make sure that you've got everything that you need. It's like checking you've got your keys, phone, cards, and whatever else you need before you head out the door. This time, you're riding off into the sunset. There's no going back, which is why you need to ensure you remember everything for change to succeed. You should know by now that achieving your weight loss goal isn't about sacrifice, struggles, hard work and diets. It's about being a good rider, motivating the elephant and smoothing the road.

RIDE INTO THE SUNSET

The Rider represents the rational thinker, the analytical planner, and the evidence-based decision-maker. The Rider can't just rely on a carefully planned and smart roadmap. The journey must appeal to the elephant's motivations, which is what a good rider does. The Rider creates a roadmap that makes sense for the elephant to follow. Even if the rider's roadmap makes sense to follow, the Elephant must be motivated to follow it. The Elephant is an emotional player full of energy, sympathy and loyalty. It moves forward, stays, or backs away based on feelings and instincts. Although the rider holds the reins and appears to lead the elephant, the six-ton beast can overpower the rider at any point. The Rider can't force the Elephant to go anywhere. Instead, the rider must motivate the Elephant in some sustainable way.

Sparks come from emotion, not from information. Once the Rider has learned how to become a good one and the Elephant is motivated, it's a case of smoothing the road that the Elephant and the Rider will follow. You need to follow the road of least resistance, and if the road is full of potholes, you need to fill them and smooth the road. If you don't, the Elephant and the Rider will have a bumpy and uncomfortable ride, inevitably giving up at some point. The last thing you need to do is check whether your roadmap is strong and you have completed everything you need for your journey to be a smooth and easy ride. You must ensure the Elephant is motivated, the Rider is a good one, and the potholes have been filled. You can't have two out of the three. You need all three to succeed. Before you ride off into the sunset, let's double-check you've got everything you need.

Is the Elephant motivated?

Without a spark of emotion, the Elephant and the Rider will be sat there with the lights on red. It would be best to have multiple feelings within you to ensure the Elephant is eager and excited to ride off in the correct direction. Do you feel slightly nervous? I'm not talking about the nerves where you doubt yourself. I'm talking about the nerves when you're just about to go and do something inspiring. The type of nerves you get before you jump out of a plane. The nerves you get before you head out on stage and sing in front of an audience. The nerves you get when you know you're going to achieve what you've always dreamed of. Before you set off on your journey, let's see if you have these feelings within you that will motivate the Elephant.

The first chapter, which centred around motivating the Elephant, was Grow Yourself. This included the three pillars: Grow Your Mindset, Improve Your Eating Habits and Be More Active. You started by working on growing your mindset, as this is where achieving anything in life begins. To motivate the Elephant, you must first believe you can lose weight. To do this, you need a growth mindset.

- Do you now have a growth mindset?
- Do you believe you can do this?

Improving your eating habits may not sound motivating to the Elephant, but it is. This is the part where you were informed that we don't diet; we eat. Learning this motivated the Elephant, as it realised it didn't have to deny itself the foods it enjoyed. This motivated the Elephant, as it didn't feel restricted and was happy with this new way of eating.

- Do you feel you can stick to this new way of eating?
- Are you happy with the new way of eating you've created?

Just like improving your eating habits, being more active doesn't sound motivating to the Elephant, but it is. The Elephant understands that it doesn't have to exercise but knows it helps to be more active. Being more active not only changes your body. It changes your mindset, your attitude, and your mood. The Elephant no longer does exercise because it has to or as a form of punishment for overeating. Instead, it is motivated to be more active because it wants to be, and when it does, it feels good for doing so.

- Have you started to be more active?
- What have you decided to do?
- How does that make you feel?

The second chapter that motivated the Elephant was Find The Feeling. You found the feeling of excitement and developed a strong emotional connection to your weight loss journey. This is where you set your goals, visualised achieving them and found something you love.

You motivated the Elephant by setting three types of goals - emotional, behavioural and motivational. Your emotional goal is your why, the deep motivating factor as to why you want to lose weight. If you don't get butterflies when you think of your why, it's not strong enough, and I encourage you to get back and rediscover your why. You also set behavioural goals that the Elephant can achieve. If you don't feel the Elephant can achieve them, shrink the behaviour so it can. Finally, you set motivational goals. It's these motivational goals that provide you with a feeling of excitement. They should provide you with enough fire in your belly to take the actions needed to go and achieve them. They aren't motivational if you do not feel excited about your goals. If this is the case, go back, rediscover, and replan your motivational goals, as they're not strong enough. It would be best to have a feeling of excitement within you to go out and achieve them.

- Have you got butterflies when thinking of your why?
- Is your why strong enough?
- When you think of your why, how does it make you feel?
- Are your behavioural goals achievable to the elephant?
- Do you have enough fire in your belly to achieve your motivational goals?
- Are you motivated to achieve your goals?

Visualising achieving your goal motivates the elephant as it brings a feeling of excitement to the table. You imagine what it feels like to achieve your goal, bringing everything to life. You visualise the journey you're about to embark on so you know what to expect, preventing the Elephant from being spooked. The Elephant has multiple feelings that motivate it to take action, as it can't wait to turn these feelings of achieving your weight loss goal into reality. I encouraged you to see progression visually by using two jars that allow you to pass every pound of weight lost into another jar, snapping monthly progress photos, or taking body measurements. You were also encouraged to get the props out, serving as daily reminders of where you're heading.

- How does it feel when you visualise achieving your weight loss goal?
- How do you feel when visualising the journey you're about to embark on?
- What does it look like?
- How have you decided to visualise your progress?
- What props have you got out to motivate you every single day?

Find Something You Love encouraged you to try new things and discover new ways of being more active. It is fun to try new things, and there's something for everyone. If you do what you love, you will enjoy it more; you will do it more. It's that simple. The Elephant will be motivated to do something if it enjoys it. Forcing the Elephant will never

work, which is why the gym doesn't get attended after two weeks. Part of your weight loss journey is to try new things, making it fun and exciting along the way.
- How many things have you tried?
- What have you tried?
- Have you found something you love that will motivate the elephant to do it regularly?

In Shrink the Change, you learned to focus on making just one change at a time. You lowered the hurdles so low that the Elephant could step over them, making change easy. This motivated the Elephant as it knew it could maintain its current pace and make gradual changes it barely noticed. You looked at what you're willing to say yes to and what you're willing to say no to. This ensured the Elephant was happy making these changes, allowing the Rider and the Elephant to be on the same page.

- Have you created a list of all the possible changes you could make?
- Have you lowered the hurdles and shrunk the change?
- Is the Elephant motivated by knowing how to make simple changes that will help you achieve this big goal of yours?

If you've done everything mentioned in this section, you've successfully motivated the Elephant, meaning the Elephant will be more than happy to follow the route set out by the Rider. There will be no resistance along your weight loss journey as the Elephant looks forward to it. It feels like this is the first time it's been considered. The energy and enthusiasm of the Elephant will fast-track your weight loss journey. Surprisingly, an Elephant can move quickly once positive emotions and feelings kick in.

Have you got control of the elephant?

The Elephant is motivated. It's eager to set off as positive feelings have been created, but you must ensure you're a good rider and have control of the Elephant. Ultimately, you want the Elephant and the Rider to work together. You don't want to force things, but you do need to control the Elephant and steer it in the right direction. If you don't, it will charge off with excitement, do doughnuts on the start line, burn itself out and have a nap. It's like releasing a balloon full of air that hasn't been tied up; You don't know where it will go. Instead, a good rider can channel the Elephant's energy to ensure it heads straight towards the true destination. Let's see if you've become a good rider and have control of the Elephant.

Bright spots ensure you follow the road of least resistance and focus on moving forward with ease. In the Find Your Bright Spots chapter, you learned to focus on the positive rather than the negative. To focus on the things you're already doing well, study them and clone them so you can do well in other areas too. Although this chapter was relatively short, it was crucial to becoming a good rider. If you follow your bright spots, you will begin your weight loss journey with no troubles.

- What are your bright spots?
- What have you learned from your bright spots?
- How have you replicated these positive actions?
- Are you focusing on moving forward with ease by following the road of least resistance?
- What would your journey look like if it was easy?

You motivated the Elephant by shrinking the change and listing many changes you could make. These were small changes, as you lowered the hurdles so low to ensure the Elephant could achieve them and wasn't spooked as it felt like it could do them. Part of being a good rider is to focus on the critical moves first. These are the ones that will have the greatest impact on your weight loss journey and fast-track you along your road. If you don't focus on your critical moves first, the Elephant will head off in the wrong direction and focus on the fancy things and the gimmicks. It will get distracted, which happens all the time. This is why the Rider is needed to ensure the changes you make are the most critical ones. You won't worry about what everyone else is doing if you're a good rider. Instead, you will be focused on your own critical moves that help you lose weight. Ensure you control the Elephant and focus on your critical moves first.

- What are your first six critical moves?

- Have you listed them in order of most significant impact?

Point To The Destination allowed the Elephant and the Rider to see which direction to head in. The first half of this chapter was Planning Ahead, which allowed the Rider to anticipate any potential barriers that may get in the way. Once you saw what may get in your way, you were encouraged to decide what you would do to overcome them. Based on your schedule, you were then asked to determine whether each week would be a weight loss week or a maintenance week. This allowed you to take the stress out of trying to lose weight during busy weeks.

- Have you anticipated any barriers that may get in your way?
- How do you plan to overcome these barriers?
- Have you prepared for the next six weeks of your weight loss journey?

The second part of Point To The Destination was where you planned your meals in a way that both the Elephant and the Rider could continue for the rest of their life. It wasn't about a diet. It was about creating a structure for each meal to ensure you were consuming the correct volumes of each food group. You understand that no food group is bad; however, the portions of each can cause you to gain weight. People tend to over-consume carbohydrates and fats but aren't consuming sufficient vegetables and proteins. With this new information, you were encouraged to plan your food consumption for each day and week, ensuring a balanced diet is consumed. Finally, you were encouraged to eat mindfully; by eating slowly, until you're satisfied rather than full, and without distractions.

- Are you consuming the correct portion sizes of each food group?
- Are you consuming the correct amount of each food group each day?
- What meal or day have you decided to improve first?
- Are you eating slowly?
- Are you eating until you're satisfied rather than full?
- Are you eating without distractions?

If you've successfully answered all of the questions in this section, you're a good rider and have control of the Elephant. Your rational and emotional thinking are intertwined to give you an unstoppable collaboration. Anything is possible when this happens, and the even better news is that you can make significant changes appear effortless. Your weight loss journey will be straightforward, and your goal will easily be achieved. You have two areas mastered, which leaves just one to check.

Have you shaped the road?

The motivated Elephant is ready to go, and the Rider has hold of the reins. The lights are on amber; however, before the lights turn green, you've got to double-check the road is straight and have put this ride in cruise control. Shape The Road was the chapter you most recently worked through, so it should still be fresh in your mind. Although it was just one chapter, it's equally as important as the three chapters centred on motivating the Elephant and the three chapters that helped you become a good rider. It's centred on creating an environment where you can flourish. It encourages you to build new habits to control your weight more easily.

The first part of Shape The Road was Tweak The Environment. Here, you considered whether you are giving yourself the best chance to lose weight and keep it off and what needs to be tweaked in your environment to make things easier. You were encouraged to build a support structure around you to ensure you have the support you need. It helps if you have people around you on your side, supporting and cheering you on every step of the way.

Unfortunately, the people you expect to help you don't support you as much as they should, which is why you need to rally the herd. Explain to them why you're doing this and how important it is for them to help you. You reviewed your sleep pattern and bedtime routine to ensure you re-energise fully each night, preventing you from using food as the primary way to energise daily. You also made your home a safe space to give you the best environment possible to succeed during your weight loss journey. You checked the kitchen cupboards and set up a workout space to ensure you live in a home that's on your side.

- Are you giving yourself the best chance to succeed on your weight loss journey?
- What needs to be tweaked in your environment?
- Do you have a strong support structure around you?
- Have you spoken to those around you to get them to help and support you every step of the way?
- Do you feel happier and at ease knowing they will be on your side?
- Are you getting enough sleep each night?
- Is your home on your side?

Building new habits was where you looked at whether your current habits are helping or hindering your progress. You were also informed how to create new habits by stacking them onto your current ones. By doing this, you can smooth out the road you're about to follow, allowing you to keep the weight off without worrying about the weight creeping back up. Building new habits is putting your journey in cruise control. You live a new lifestyle that you enjoy, meaning you no longer worry or think about your weight creeping up as you know these new actions control your weight without ever having to think about them.

- Are your current habits helping or hindering your progress?
- Which current habit are you going to begin stacking on top of?
- What new habits will you choose to stack?

If you can successfully answer every question I've asked, you've successfully Shaped The Road, have control of the Elephant, and have motivated the Elephant too. The road is now clear, and the lights are ready to change. The Elephant and the Rider are relaxed, yet excited. The sun is shining, and it's time for them to put their sunglasses on, select their favourite songs, and embark on their journey together. Like creating a playlist of your favourite songs before setting off on your journey, you need to put everything you've learned and planned into a simple weekly format. I call this your weight loss roadmap.

CREATE YOUR WEIGHT LOSS ROADMAP

If you've been using this book correctly and are serious about losing weight for good, you should have one of two things by now. One: Lots of pieces of paper with your notes for each chapter. Two: a notepad containing all the notes you've written while working your way through the book. If you haven't, then although I praise you for reading my book until the very end, and I hope you enjoyed it and found it helpful, what on earth have you been doing? This book is about action. Without the information from the to-do list of each chapter, you can't create your weight loss roadmap.

Visit The Weight Loss Academy's website at www.theweightlossacademy.com/roadmap. Here, you will find a download for you to print off. You will use this document each week to create your own weight loss roadmap. Grab all your notes, as you need them to map out your journey.

I've kept this document as simple as possible, as I know you're busy. You only need to spend a minute or two each day on this sheet. You should have planned half the things on here in advance, from the Script The Critical Moves and Point To The Destination chapters. The rest is logging what you've done each week. All the information I cover refers to the roadmap download you will find on the website. It would be a good idea to download this document now, as this section will instruct you on how to use it so you can create your weight loss roadmap. Once again, this document is found at www.theweightlossacademy.com/roadmap.

Section One: Find your notes from the Point To The Destination Chapter; you should have written down any potential barriers for each week over the next six weeks. Write down your potential barrier for each week on your roadmap sheet next to 'Potential Barriers'. Underneath, it says 'What's The Plan?', write down how you plan to overcome these barriers. Based on your potential barriers for each week, you must decide whether it's a weight loss or maintenance week. Where it says 'Lose or Maintain?', write down whether it's a weight loss week or a maintenance week.

Find your notes from the Script The Critical Moves Chapter; you should have a list of your critical moves. I asked you to put your critical moves in order of the greatest impact. Then, on a scale of 1-10, you asked yourself how consistent you could be with each critical move. It has to be a nine or ten out of ten for you to focus on making the change. If it's any lower, don't make it right now. Where it says 'My Critical Move Is', write down your weekly critical move. Week one should be the most critical, impacting your weight loss journey the most. Remember, only write it on your roadmap if you can be consistent with this change. One critical move doesn't have to be made each week. If you need more time to make it, write down the same critical move in the next week.

Find your notes from the Track Your Food Intake Chapter. Using My Fitness Pal, you discover the number of daily calories to consume if it's a weight loss week and the amount if it's a maintenance week. Depending on which type of week it is, next to 'Weekly Calorie Total', write down the number of weekly calories you can consume. For example, if it's 1500 calories per day, multiply it by seven to equal 10,500.

You decide how you distribute your calories throughout the week. Not every week is the same. This is why it's important to track how many calories you've consumed each day, along with how many calories you have left remaining for the week. Underneath 'Weekly Calorie Total' is a table. At the end of each day write down how many calories you've consumed that day in the calories column. In the remaining column, write down how many calories you have remaining for the week. Section one ensures you know what each week entails, how you plan to stay on track, how many calories you aim to consume this week, and how many calories you're consuming each day.

Section Two: This section is about tracking a range of things. The first is the consistency of your critical moves. Underneath each day of the week, place a tick if you've managed to be consistent with your critical move. If you haven't, place a cross in the box. 80% consistent would be six out of seven days. That's where you need to be before you move on to your next critical move.

The next five rows are all about the food and drink you consume daily. The purpose of this book is to encourage you to discover a sustainable way of eating that will help you lose weight and keep it off. Yes, it's centred around weight loss; however, I want you to thrive and be full of energy. Not to forget, to allow your body to function correctly. To do this, you need to ensure most of your food intake is from smart food choices. In row two, write down the number of fruits and vegetables you've eaten each day. In row three, write down the number of smart proteins you've eaten. In row four write down the number of smart fats you've eaten. In row five, write down the number of smart carbohydrates you've eaten. Row six is where you track how many glasses of water you're consuming each day. These rows allow you to see progress being made as, over time, you will see the numbers increase.

Sleep is essential as it's the body's primary method of re-energising. Sufficient sleep ensures you won't search for sugary foods to increase your energy levels throughout the day, which increases your calorie intake. If you sleep better, you will eat better; it's that simple. In row seven, you're asked how much sleep you had each evening. Place the number of hours in each day of the week. This allows you to review your sleep duration and see if there is a link between lack of sleep and calories consumed.

Continuing on from re-energising, row eight is a place to track your energy levels. If you're eating smart foods and are sleeping well, you should feel energised. On this row, rate your energy levels on a scale of one to ten. Place a low number if you're low on energy and place a high number if you're full of beans.

Row nine tracks the difficulty of each day. How difficult has it been to stick to your plan today? If it has been a smooth sailing day, place a low number. If it has been way too tricky, place a high number. If the numbers are high, take five minutes to think about whether you're trying to do too much at once. If things feel too difficult, lower the hurdle even lower by shrinking the changes you're trying to make.

Row ten is all about your emotions. Remember, it's best to notice and name how you feel, as your emotions dictate your direction. This section ensures your feelings are positive and the Elephant is motivated. If things feel too hard, restrictive, tiring, or any other negative feeling, the Elephant will run off in the wrong direction. Rate your emotions on a scale of one to ten. If you're feeling super positive, place a high number. If you're feeling ok, place a middle number. If you have negative emotions, place a low number.

Finally, row eleven is a place to track your activity levels. You can do this in one of two ways. The first option is to tick the box on the days you exercise. The other option is to place the duration of each exercise session in the box. It's your roadmap so do whichever option suits you.

Section Three: The final section of your roadmap is your weekly evaluation. This section can be found at the bottom left of the page. Here, you're encouraged to reflect on your week and discover what you have done well this week, what you found challenging, and how you can improve the following week. Reflection is such a valuable tool to use in your life. It allows you to stop and think about your own behaviours. If you're doing well, it's a fantastic way to take a little time to praise yourself. If things aren't working well for you, it's the perfect moment to stop and plan your next move.

The first part of reflection is 'What Have I Done Well', where you write down all of the things you've done well this week and are happy with. This section motivates the Elephant by discovering bright spots throughout your journey. These could be physical achievements, sticking to your changes, or feeling more positive or energised.

The second reflection section is "What I Found Challenging'. This is where you write down the parts of your week, activities, or changes you found challenging. The goal is for this section to remain clear most of the time as your roadmap should be simple to follow. There are many potential reasons you find your week challenging, such as not having enough time to exercise, difficulty juggling work and social life, or the chocolate was calling your name all week.

The third reflection section is 'How I Can Improve Next Week'. Ultimately, this is why you reflect on things; to use your growth mindset and look at ways of self-improvement. If you found it challenging to stick to your changes, shrink the change. If you were tempted by chocolate all week, could you factor in some dark chocolate into next week? If you didn't have much time to exercise, could you reduce the duration and frequency but increase the intensity?

The goal of reflection is to praise yourself for the things you're doing well, allowing you to discover further bright spots in your life that you can investigate and clone for further success. Reflection encourages you to think about what you found challenging, so you can shrink the change to allow the road to weight loss to be simple to follow. Finally, it stimulates the growth mindset by continually looking at ways of improving yourself. All of this comes together to motivate the Elephant and improve as the Rider.

That is your weekly roadmap explained. This may sound like a lot to do, but you've already planned half of it. The other half is keeping tabs on other things and writing a number in a box daily. It takes two seconds out of your day. Some sections may sound a little silly, but you should understand the importance of your emotions and feelings. Don't be embarrassed to write or talk about your feelings. Instead, reflect on your feelings and review your days and week's performance to feel happier, be more content, and allow your weight loss journey to be smoother and more enjoyable.

When you look at your weekly roadmap, it's just a piece of paper with boxes and words on it. To many, it doesn't seem like much, but that's the point, it isn't. It's supposed to be a daily and weekly habit that's easy to do. Remember, any new habit change should take less than five minutes to complete. Completing your roadmap takes less than five minutes out of your week. When you take a minute, you will see the true power of your weight loss roadmap.

Your weekly roadmap fused with MyFitnessPal ensures you're on the road to weight loss. Tracking your food intake via MyFitnessPal is essential when you're on your weight loss journey. It's also important to continue tracking your food intake once you achieve your weight loss goal. You will need to learn the volume of food you can consume to the calories as your weekly calorie intake will be higher to maintain weight.

I've now provided you with all the information and structure needed to succeed on your weight loss journey. This book is my creation; however, what's been produced by this book is yours. By following everything in this book, one chapter at a time, you've created a weight loss roadmap for yourself. This means it will work for you and fit into your lifestyle. You will be happy to follow it because you created it. You will look forward to your meals as you've chosen what to eat. You have created your motivating factors. The changes you're going to make have been chosen by you. You get the idea. Each person who has read this book starts at the same point and will finish with the same goal of getting to their target weight, but the true beauty of this book is everyone's journey is unique to them.

When people see your amazing weight loss success, they will ask how you did it. This question leads to "What diet have you been following?" which is the adult term for "Can I copy your homework?". They want to save themselves the time and energy of finding a way of losing weight for themselves. They see you as the guinea pig and know your way works. This is why they want to copy you; however, it won't work for them. This is because you have created your own way of losing weight. When people copy, they don't think about the best way for themselves to lose weight. For them to successfully lose weight, they need to create their own weight loss roadmap. They need to discover a way that's going to work for them.

If anybody asks, tell them to read this book 'The Road To Weight Loss: Create Your Roadmap To Weight Loss Success'. This way, they will be recommended something that works, and you will gain kudos for your excellent results. Ideally, tell them to buy their own copy rather than lend it to them so I can make a living, but there is no harm in a bit of book sharing. I wrote this book to spread a message and help as many people as possible achieve their weight loss goals. If you enjoyed the book and know the structure within it works, tell everyone. You have the power not only to change your life but also to show others there's a way of losing weight that will help them too. It's important to spread the word and get as many people as possible out of the diet trap. People can change their lives for the better, and you can be the beginning of that change for them.

It's funny how the end of a book can also be the beginning. You've created your weight loss roadmap; however, you're at the beginning of the road to weight loss. You've built a support structure around you. Yet, my job wouldn't be complete if I didn't create a place for each person who reads this book to share their trials and tribulations, success stories and tips they've learnt along the way. A special community of people who made it to their target weight or are following their road to weight loss. It's each person's role to help others in life, and you can do this by becoming a Weight Loss Academy member. As a member, you will gain access to our weight loss forum, weight loss support groups, and monthly workshops. The more people contributing to the weight loss forum, the stronger your support structure will be. Although each person is following their own road to weight loss, we can feel as though we are in this together. Each person is on a weight loss journey which is why we can support one another every step of the way. Become a member at www.theweightlossacademy.com/join.

Finally, the Weight Loss Academy is more than this book. It's our job to ensure as many people as possible achieve their weight loss goals. It begins with this book, however, we also help others create their weight loss roadmap through our weight loss course, The Road To Weight Loss. If you have read this book, but feel as though an interactive course led by a weight loss coach would help, take a look at the next available course dates at www.theweightlossacademy.com/course.

We also offer private weight loss coaching and mentoring. If, at any point throughout your weight loss journey, you feel as though you require additional support, either become a weight loss academy member or book a weight loss coaching call. You can find further information about our weight loss coaching services on our website at www.theweightlossacademy.com/coaching.

I've officially covered everything you need to succeed on your weight loss journey. The sun is shining on your face. The day is coming to a close. The Rider knows where they're going. It's the first time you've ever embarked on a weight loss journey, and felt calm and confident as you've mapped out the journey ahead. The Elephant is motivated to follow the road you've created as it knows it will not be mistreated. Instead, your deep motivating factor and 'Why' will fuel the Elephant to follow the road to weight loss and travel towards your destination. Gone are the cloudy days. It's time to put one foot in front of the other and leave the restrictive days behind. It feels good knowing what's ahead—times of achievement, positive emotions, and content. You will never have to diet or try to lose weight ever again. It's time for you to follow the road to weight loss and ride off into the sunset. I wish you good luck and farewell

Useful Links

Roadmap Download
www.theweightlossacademy.com/roadmap

Become A Weight Loss Academy Member
www.theweightlossacademy.com/join

Book On Our Next Course
www.theweightlossacademy.com/weightlosscourse

Hire A Weight Loss Coach
www.theweightlossacademy.com/weightlosscoaching